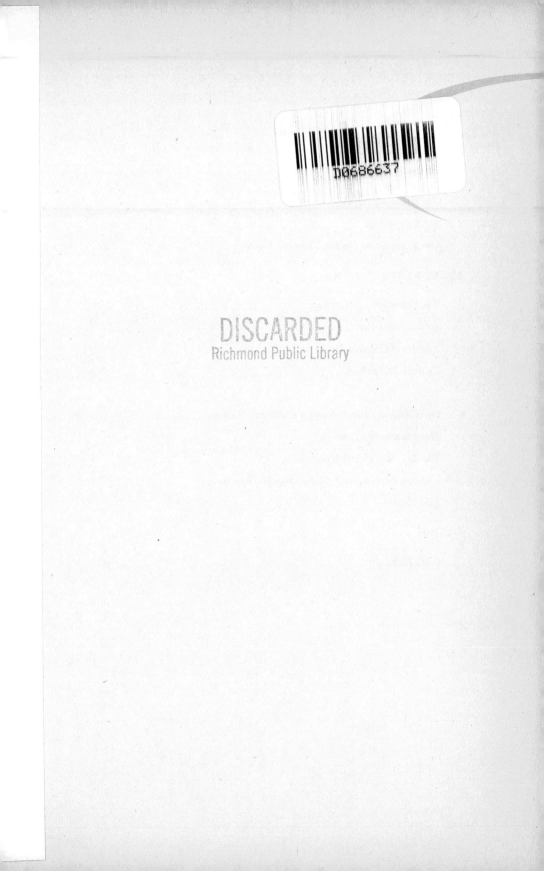

BOOKS EDITED BY LEE GUTKIND

Connecting

The Essayist at Work

Surviving Crisis

Our Roots Grow Deeper Than We Know

BOOKS BY LEE GUTKIND

The Veterinarian's Touch

An Unspoken Art

The Art of Creative Nonfiction

Creative Nonfiction

Stuck in Time

One Children's Place: Inside a Children's Hospital

Many Sleepless Nights

The People of Penn's Woods West

The Best Seat in Baseball, But You Have to Stand!

Bike Fever

FICTION

God's Helicopter

healing

TWENTY PROMINENT AUTHORS

WRITE ABOUT INSPIRATIONAL

MOMENTS OF ACHIEVING HEALTH

AND GAINING INSIGHT

edited by lee gutkind

JEREMY P. TARCHER/PUTNAM
A MEMBER OF PENGUIN PUTNAM INC.
NEW YORK

Most Tarcher/Putnam books are available at special quantity discounts for bulk purchase for sales promotions, premiums, fund-raising, and educational needs. Special books or book excerpts also can be created to fit specific needs. For details, write Putnam Special Markets, 375 Hudson Street, New York, NY 10014.

Jeremy P. Tarcher/Putnam
a member of
Penguin Putnam Inc.
375 Hudson Street
New York, NY 10014
www.penguinputnam.com

Library of Congress Cataloging-in-Publication Data

Healing : twenty prominent authors write about inspirational moments
of achieving health and gaining insight / edited by Lee Gutkind.
p.   cm.
ISBN 1-58542-079-4
1. Health—Miscellanea.   2. Health—Literary collections.
3. Healing—Literary collections.   I. Gutkind, Lee.

RA776.5 .H37   2001   00-048887
610—dc21

Printed in the United States of America

1   3   5   7   9   10   8   6   4   2

BOOK DESIGN BY RALPH L. FOWLER

acknowledgments

I wish to thank Patricia Park and Coral Ruppert of *Creative Nonfiction* magazine for their assistance in the preparation of this collection—and Irene Prokop for its inspiration.

contents

healing

the rope test

a magic moment

When I was a teenager, my mother always assured me that I wasn't fat; rather, I was big boned. And I had a very slow metabolism. Both observations were probably true, but not the main reason I weighed 220 pounds (my suit size 44 [Husky] when I graduated high school)—too fat for the marines or the air force. I assumed that by enlisting in the U.S. Coast Guard, the only service that would accept me at my weight, I would have an easy time of it, physically. After all, they were the shallow-water sailors. Little did I know that because we were operating mostly on the coast (guarding our shores from enemy aggression), we would always be running like hell.

A favorite drill in basic training (boot camp) was triggered by a certain signal on the bell tower—three staccato chimes. At that moment, we recruits, wherever we were standing, whatever we were doing, were obliged to grab our pieces (M1 rifles) and bayonets and dash to meet an invading enemy and do combat in the water. Traditional coast guard boot camp was twelve weeks versus the army's nine-week stint. But even after twelve weeks of basic, I was the only member of my company not allowed to graduate and join a unit. I had lost a good deal of weight at this point—and was certainly as fit as I had ever been—having been forced to march endlessly, do hundreds of push-ups and sit-ups each day, and run and dive maniacally through the U.S. Marine–style obstacle course. But I could not seem to pass the rope test. This was a rope, fifty feet high, with knots spaced evenly for handholds; you needed to climb to the top and then control your descent. There were other ways of boarding an invading ship, but if a rope was the only answer, a coast guardsman must be able to do it. Every night after supper, I was tested, and every night I failed.

During the day I worked with a maintenance crew inside an abandoned boiler, chiseling away at the burnt-in soot and debris for hours on end without seeing natural light between breakfast and lunch and lunch and supper. At that time, masks were unheard of. You breathed in the coal dust in the morning and coughed it out at night. By day's end, I lacked the energy and determination to climb the rope or even to work out with free weights to strengthen my upper body. Not wanting to remain in boot-camp limbo for the rest of my hitch, I started to get up early in the morning and do hundreds of push-ups and sit-ups before reveille. At lunch, instead of eating or smoking, I would take long walks around the compound. Or I went into the men's room and practiced pull-ups on the toilet stall doors. The guys with whom I shared boiler-cleaning duty were in detention because of some criminal act they had committed and not because they were too fat or couldn't pass the rope test. They would not have taken kindly to my "public" display of extra physical training. Their attitude was that we had plenty enough P.T. in our own routine.

Under my secret regimen, however, no more than ten days went by before I surprised myself and my instructors by literally bounding up the rope from floor to ceiling, which I touched with one sure hand, then skittered down again without using my feet. When I got to the bottom the first time, I showboated by going up again—and back. It was a triumphant moment, not just because I succeeded, but more so because of the ease with which I pulled it off.

A few years later, I realized that my struggle to climb the ropes as a coast guard recruit—and my eventual success—symbolized a rare and precious breakthrough. Up to that point, I had understood the work ethic, but suddenly the possibilities and potential of my life were much more evident than ever before. For years, I had felt trapped by a nervous and voracious hunger and the negative body image it had created. My nickname, which triggered my humiliation and my fists, was Slim. My mother had always assured me that fatness was in my genes, that it had little to do with exercise or eating habits. But now, I suddenly discovered, I could be in control. I remember returning home on my first leave after basic training—permitted after passing the rope test—and approaching my anxious mother, waiting at the bus station. I stopped a few feet in front of her, spread my arms to embrace her and . . . she walked right by me!

"You don't recognize your own son?" I said.

She turned and looked as if she had never seen me before and then began to cry. "Oh my God, what have they done to my child?" she squealed.

I remember wanting to tell her not what they had done to me, but what the military had done *for* me. I wanted to recount that magic moment on the summit of the rope when I suddenly realized my own potential as a human being, that I could be self-reliant and feel safe in my own hands. Instead, I smiled, patted her shoulders reassuringly, and explained that I was feeling fine. I was the same beloved son she had kissed good-bye five months before—just sixty pounds lighter. I knew that neither she nor anyone else would understand what had changed me and how intense or overwhelming that change would turn out to be. Few barriers (emotional or physical) would ever stop me from achieving the goals I truly longed for. Not many months later, I began to write—a dream I had secretly harbored for most of my life, which I now realized was within my grasp.

. . .

Although the overall theme is health (wellness and sickness, etc.), most essays in *Healing* contain a "magic" healing moment. Some of these moments are more evident than others, as in Lucy Grealy's epiphany during dinner with her handsome young man, or Leonard Kriegel's fall on Fourteenth Street and his acknowledgment of a need for help. Other moments come as complete surprises, such as the sudden introduction of Dr. Van Skeldt in "Night Rhythms," which changes the entire thrust of the narrative, or when Susan Adkins's sister, impersonating their father, doffs her wig.

For the most part, the magic moments in these essays symbolize or conceptualize healing, but it is important to point out that most of the best essays ever written, whatever the subject, will usually contain a moment, however fleeting, when divergent elements—plot, scene, characters, informational aspects—touch and blend. That moment should trigger a memorable burst of clarity and recognition that will remain forever vivid for both writer and reader. Look for those moments in *Healing*. Think of an essay as a story that somewhere, somehow, contains a moment when a hidden area is suddenly illuminated, and a bright yellow swath of recognition and connection explodes across the page.

carol sanford

Although rich with devices, Carol Sanford's essay is crisp and unadorned. She employs a ruddy gold blanket as a vehicle to mark the passing of time, along with her journal, which effectively captures her present-day life. The tragic death of her son is announced with simple clarity. She and her husband rebuild their life with the building of a log cabin serving as an effective metaphor. Her magic moment arrives when her son is enveloped in the cosmos—and she is able to finally let him go.

bed, blanket, window

It's morning. Before I open my eyes in the loft of our unheated log cabin, I feel chilly September air teasing my nose. The cabin smells of new pine. I am warm lying beside my husband, Glenn, under a fifty-year-old wool blanket whose color I've always thought of as burnt gold. This is a blanket that knows my history.

When I lived under my parents' roof, my bedroom was in the attic, where no heat warmed the air in winter unless the stairway door stayed open. I shared that room with my older sister. The walls were unfinished knotty-pine boards, and between our built-in twin beds, a small window opened out onto the world. What I saw from there most evenings was a sunset that bled trails of purple, pink, and orange above the flat farmland to the west and north. That view made me sure I wanted to be a writer, but writing was hard work in a frigid room. Mom bought full-sized, thick wool blankets from Montgomery Ward and put them on our beds. My sister's green blanket seemed more desirable to me than mine, which was burnt gold—a shade or two darker than my topaz birthstone ring. I had a sense that the green and gold symbolized the different lives my sister and I would lead, and perhaps green was exactly right for her; she has lived a life of considerable happiness, harmony, and financial well-being.

Some time would pass before I could know what burnt gold might mean for me.

Glenn and I are in the long process of building this cabin. Every-

where you look you feel warmed inside by the soft glow of pine logs and boards, which I have spent much of the summer sanding and sealing. We sleep on an air mattress, our temporary bed, which we've positioned directly under a skylight that opens. This strange window, bordered by pine rafters and horizontal tongue-and-groove knotty pine, offers us one view: up. Some nights it is a mirror for love-making as well as an invitation to the night. Stars appear, as if to us alone, through the dark silhouettes of oak leaves.

Over the years, I learned to appreciate the warmth of my blanket; I hated to crawl out from under it on frosty mornings to dress, although I loved school. There I made friends easily, gregariously, yet at home I was a quiet, sensitive child. Heavy abuse of alcohol in our household caused me to spend hours in my room where the best coping mechanisms I could come up with were reading and keeping a diary in which I laid out weekly plans for self-improvement (longer study hours, better grades, weight loss, Bible reading, prayers before bed). The subtext was always the family secret. My inner life, constantly burnished by painful emotion, became very important to me.

But there in my room, under the blanket, far more than downstairs with my family or at school, I felt comfortable with my changing, bleeding body. Beneath its weight I could ponder and worry about other things, like sex. There I could pretend to feel the would-be babies inside me as I lay curled like a fetus to conserve body heat. They were invisible beings safe in my belly, and only a few of them would be born. I wanted four children, like my mother who had achieved the perfect symmetry of two girls and then two boys.

Last night we lay here tired after long hours of hard work, content to recount the day's accomplishments and make a verbal list of all the things we will do today: begin the ceramic tile project, apply polyurethane to the cedar trim intended for the kitchen windows, move some black dirt from down by the river to next spring's strawberry patch, put an extra coat of water repellent on the deck because winter is coming.

My gold blanket went with me to college, where it lay at the foot of more than one bunk bed in more than one shoe-box-size room, and on into marriage. Then for several years it stayed at the back of an attic closet in the home my first husband and I built in the country to raise our family. There I slept in a second-story bedroom with a view of sky and picturesque trees. I covered our bed with the popular look—a fuzzy, olive green spread. By then, at twenty-five, I'd had two boys and a girl, and three seemed enough even though I thrived on being a mother. When our daughter was still in diapers we began to spend part of every August camped on Lake Charlevoix in northwest Michigan, and the blanket came in handy.

I decided to launder it myself after several summers because I felt that dry cleaning would be too expensive. I suppose I didn't really care if it was ruined; I still had reservations about the color, and I didn't like its rough texture either. The blanket was limp when I pulled it from the washing machine and lugged it to the clothesline, but its deep gold-brown remained intact. I didn't throw it out, even though I preferred that things look bright and glossy in those days—including my marriage. There, an old emptiness was multiplying itself, until finally I had to acknowledge the anguish of a failed relationship, and then live with it. I followed the lead of women in my family, who bear their sorrows silently.

That marriage lasted for twenty-three years and when I left, the blanket went with me. It was truly mine, preceding all joint ownership and older than two other such items I took along: a Samsonite suitcase and a manual Smith Corona typewriter, both high school graduation presents. For the next two years I kept these things in the basement of the apartment building I lived in, and there the blanket picked up a large mildew stain I was never able to get out. I slept in a twin-size bed on the first floor of the building, where my bedroom window looked out on city traffic. In many ways I was lucky, but that period of being single—carrying the stigma of divorce and living alone for the first time in my life—was a time of agony. My days were full of the friction of guilt versus right path, of old values versus true values, of the wife-mother role versus the role of a new woman. I was in such pain I couldn't have guessed that the trial by fire was yet to come . . .

Some mornings when I wake, even here in this haven, even three years and more after the accident, my first realization is that my child is dead. Other mornings I am conscious of it before I wake, and that's somehow better. I'm less inclined to be physically aware of my womb's emptiness, how it gapes like a crater carved by hard shock. Yes, my second son, my middle child, is gone.

This man beside me—my second husband and soul mate—stirs now. I lie still so he'll rest a few minutes longer. A light sleeper, he wakes often in the night to remember his dreams and listen to me breathe.

The sudden death of your child stops everything. You hear the terrible news, become enveloped in protective shock, and wake up later unable to grasp how you are to go on living. For me, time's passage meant nothing. Clocks inferred madness—*tick, tick, tick*—or Chinese water torture: *plop . . . plop . . . plop . . . plop. . . .* The hangman's hood had come down over my head quickly, and I could see nothing as I waited in numbness for my own death.

We helped save ourselves by buying land with trees and a river running the length of it. My husband's long-standing dream was to build a log cabin, and at fifty-four he felt the time had come. But we didn't rush into construction. With the death of a loved one you learn in a new way that a rich, evolving process matters far more than the end product. How you live is more critical than how, or even when, you die.

We first canoed the river and played in the pine forest like children pretending to set up housekeeping. We became acquainted with the deer and wild turkeys. We took down a dead cherry tree and transplanted small spruce and pine to sunnier spots. We created a memorial of wood and stone for my son. Then we devoted many months to building the garage we would need to store our tools and materials for building the cabin. We sided the garage with rough-sawed lumber, taking pains to cut and match the boards for an artistic effect and staining them the color we'd chosen for the log cabin—a classic rusty hue. Finally, after three summers, the cabin went up.

Last night I got out the burnt gold blanket and studied it as I unfolded it over our bed. It's a bit limp yet still coarse in texture, stained but still bold with color. The dark brown stitching along the edges is raveling badly, but I'll repair it soon. I like the weight of this blanket on my bones.

If the blanket tells me where I've been, this window above moves me to a new place. Just as I once imagined my would-be children safe inside me, I now imagine my again invisible son out there, safe in the belly of the cosmos. He has come here, and gone, but sometimes I am wonderfully connected. Through the skylight, I see my child walking a lane that spirals somewhere in the universe. He is happy, yet contemplating coming back to earth for more experience. Here, he can resume accumulating what his spirit needs, all spirits need, to continue expanding: knowledge, awareness, love. He will have another mother, a different body, another life. I can let him go . . . Just now it strikes me I may always have known that to be burnished within by living—again and again, until we glow golden—is the point of it all.

Under the blanket I touch my husband's shoulder to let him know I'm awake. It's time for us to get up. We have many things to do.

lucy grealy

"Mirrorings" is especially effective because of a specificity of focus: Grealy's emotional trauma in relation to her face and the process of healing. She steers clear of those aspects of her life that are not directly related. The essay is also informative. The reader learns a great deal about plastic surgery and the lingering effects of serious illness long after recovery. Here, the magic healing moment with her handsome dinner companion becomes a powerful metaphor of her triumph.

mirrorings

There was a long period of time, almost a year, during which I never looked in a mirror. It wasn't easy, for I'd never suspected just how omnipresent are our own images. I began by merely avoiding mirrors, but by the end of the year I found myself with an acute knowledge of the reflected image, its numerous tricks and wiles, how it can spring up at any moment: a glass tabletop, a well-polished door handle, a darkened window, a pair of sunglasses, a restaurant's otherwise magnificent brass-plated coffee machine sitting innocently by the cash register.

At the time, I had just moved, alone, to Scotland and was surviving on the dole, as Britain's social security benefits are called. I didn't know anyone and had no idea how I was going to live, yet I went anyway because by happenstance I'd met a plastic surgeon there who said he could help me. I had been living in London, working temp jobs. While in London, I'd received more nasty comments about my face than I had in the previous three years, living in Iowa, New York, and Germany. These comments, all from men and all odiously sexual, hurt and disoriented me. I also had journeyed to Scotland because after more than a dozen operations in the States my insurance had run out, along with my hope that further operations could make any *real* difference. Here, however, was a surgeon who had some new techniques, and here, amazingly enough, was a government willing to foot the bill: I didn't feel I could pass up yet another chance to "fix" my face, which I confusedly thought would be concurrent with "fixing" my self, my soul, my life.

. . .

Twenty years ago, when I was nine and living in America, I came home from school one day with a toothache. Several weeks and misdiagnoses later, surgeons removed most of the right side of my jaw in an attempt to prevent the cancer they found there from spreading. No one properly explained the operation to me, and I awoke in a cocoon of pain that prevented me from moving or speaking. Tubes ran in and out of my body, and because I was temporarily unable to speak after the surgery and could not ask questions, I made up my own explanations for the tubes' existence. I remember the mysterious manner the adults displayed toward me. They asked me to do things: lie still for X rays, not cry for needles, and so on, tasks that, although not easy, never seemed equal to the praise I received in return. Reinforced to me again and again was how I was "a brave girl" for not crying, "a good girl" for not complaining, and soon I began defining myself this way, equating strength with silence.

Then the chemotherapy began. In the seventies chemo was even cruder than it is now, the basic premise being to poison patients right up to the very brink of their own death. Until this point I almost never cried and almost always received praise in return. Thus I got what I considered the better part of the deal. But now it was like a practical joke that had gotten out of hand. Chemotherapy was a nightmare and I wanted it to stop; I didn't want to be brave anymore. Yet I had grown so used to defining myself as brave, as *silent,* that the thought of losing this sense of myself was even more terrifying. I was certain that if I broke down I would be despicable in the eyes of both my parents and the doctors.

The task of taking me into the city for the chemo injections fell mostly on my mother, though sometimes my father made the trip. Overwhelmed by the sight of the vomiting and weeping, my father developed the routine of "going to get the car," meaning that he left the doctor's office before the injection was administered, on the premise that then he could have the car ready and waiting when it was all over. Ashamed of my suffering, I felt relief when he was finally out of the room. When my mother took me, she stayed in the room, yet this only made the distance between us even more tangible. She explained that it was wrong to cry *before* the needle went in; afterward was one thing, but before, that was mere fear, and hadn't I demonstrated my bravery earlier? Every Friday for two and a half years I climbed up onto that big doctor's table and told myself not to cry, and every week I failed. The two large syringes were filled with chemicals so caustic to the vein that each had to be administered very slowly. The whole process took about four minutes; I had to remain utterly still. Dry retching began in the first fifteen seconds, then the throb behind my eyes gave everything a yellow-green aura, and the bone-deep pain of alternating extreme hot and cold flashes made me tremble, yet still I had to sit motionless and not move my arm. No one spoke to me—not the doctor, who was a paradigm of the cold-fish physician; not the nurse, who told my mother I reacted much more violently than many of "the other children"; and not my mother, who, surely over-whelmed by the sight of her child's suffering, thought the best thing to do was remind me to be brave, to try not to cry. All the while I hated myself for having wept before the needle went in, convinced that the nurse and my mother were right, that I was "overdoing it," that the throwing up was phychosomatic, that my mother was angry with me for not being good or brave enough.

Yet each week, two or three days after the injection, there came the first flicker of feeling better, the always forgotten and gratefully rediscovered understanding that to simply be well in my body was the greatest thing I could ask for. I thought other people felt this appreciation and physical joy all the time, and I felt cheated because I was able to feel it only once a week.

Because I'd lost my hair, I wore a hat constantly, but this fooled no one, least of all myself. During this time, my mother worked in a nursing home in a Hasidic community. Hasidic law dictates that married women cover their hair, and most commonly this is done with a wig. My mother's friends were now all too willing to donate their discarded wigs, and soon the house seemed filled with them. I never wore one, for they frightened me even when my mother insisted I looked better in one of the few that actually fit. Yet we didn't know how to say no to the women who kept graciously offering their wigs. The cats enjoyed sleeping on them and the dogs playing with them, and we grew used to having to pick a wig up off a chair we wanted to sit in. It never struck us as odd until one day a visitor commented wryly as he cleared a chair for himself, and suddenly a great wave of shame overcame me. I had nightmares about wigs and flushed if I even heard the word, and one night I put myself out of my misery by getting up after everyone was asleep and gathering all the wigs except for one the dogs were fond of and that they had chewed up anyway. I hid all the rest in an old chest.

When you are only ten, which is when the chemotherapy began, two and a half years seem like your whole life, yet it did finally end, for the cancer was gone. I remember the last day of treatment clearly because it was the only day on which I succeeded in not crying, and because later, in private, I cried harder than I had in years; I thought now I would no longer be "special," that without the arena of chemotherapy in which to prove myself no one would ever love me, that I would fade unnoticed into the background. But this idea about *not being different* didn't last very long. Before, I foolishly believed that people stared at me because I was bald. After my hair eventually grew in, it didn't take long before I understood that I looked different for another reason. My face. People stared at me in stores, and other children made fun of me to the point that I came to expect such reactions constantly, wherever I went. School became a battleground.

Halloween, that night of frights, became my favorite holiday because I could put on a mask and walk among the blessed for a few brief, sweet hours. Such freedom I felt, walking down the street, my face hidden! Through the imperfect oval holes I could peer out at other faces, masked or painted or not, and see on those faces nothing but the normal faces of childhood looking back at me, faces I mistakenly thought were the faces everyone else but me saw all the time, faces that were simply curious and ready for fun, not the faces I usually braced myself for, the cruel, lonely, vicious ones I spent every day other than Halloween waiting to see around each corner. As I breathed in the condensed, plastic-scented air under the mask, I somehow thought that I was breathing in normality, that this joy and weightlessness were what the world was composed of, and that it was only my face that kept me from it, my face that was my own mask and kept me from knowing the joy I was sure everyone but me lived with intimately. How could the other children not know it? Not know that to be free of the fear of taunts and the burden of knowing no one would ever love you was all that anyone could ask for? I was a pauper walking for a short while in the clothes of the prince, and when the day ended I gave up my disguise with dismay.

I was living in an extreme situation, and because I did not particularly care for the world I was in, I lived in others, and because the world I did live in was dangerous now, I incorporated this danger into my secret life. I imagined myself to be an Indian. Walking down the streets, I stepped through the forest, my body ready for any opportunity to fight or flee one of the big cats that I knew stalked me. Vietnam and Cambodia, in the news then as scenes of catastrophic horror, were other places I walked through daily. I made my way down the school hall, knowing a land mine or a sniper might give themselves away at any moment with the subtle metal click I'd read about. Compared with a land mine, a mere insult about my face seemed a frivolous thing.

In those years, not yet a teenager, I secretly read—knowing it was somehow inappropriate—works by Primo Levi and Elie Wiesel, and every book by a survivor I could find by myself without asking the librarian. Auschwitz, Birkenau: I felt the blows of the *capos* and somehow knew that because at any moment we might be called upon to live for a week on one loaf of bread and some water called soup, the peanut butter sandwich I found on my plate was nothing less than a miracle, an utter and sheer miracle capable of making me literally weep with joy.

I decided to become a "deep" person. I wasn't exactly sure what this would entail, but I believed that if I could just find the right philosophy, think the right thoughts, my suffering would end. To try to understand the world I was in, I undertook to find out what was "real," and I quickly began seeing reality as existing in the lowest common denominator, that suffering was the one and only dependable thing. But rather than spend all of my time despairing, though certainly I did plenty of that, I developed a form of defensive egomania: I felt I was the only one walking about in a world who understood what was really important. I looked upon people complaining about the most mundane things—nothing on TV, traffic jams, the price of new clothes—and felt joy because I knew how unimportant those things really were and felt unenlightened superiority because other people didn't. Because in my fantasy life I had learned to be thankful for each cold, blanketless night that I survived on the cramped wooden bunks, my pain and despair were a stroll though the country in comparison. I was often miserable, but I knew that to feel warm instead of cold was its own kind of joy, that to eat was a reenactment of the grace of some god whom I could only dimly define, and that to simply be alive was a rare, ephemeral gift.

As I became a teenager, my isolation began. My nonidentical twin sister started going out with boys, and I started—my most tragic mistake of all—to listen to and believe the taunts thrown at me daily by the very boys she and the other girls were interested in. I was a dog, a monster, the ugliest girl they had ever seen. Of all the remarks, the most damaging wasn't even directed at me but was really an insult to "Jerry," a boy I never saw because every day between fourth and fifth periods, when I was cornered by a particular group of kids, I was too ashamed to lift my eyes off the floor. "Hey, look, it's Jerry's girlfriend!" they shrieked when they saw me, and I felt such shame, knowing that this was the deepest insult to Jerry that they could imagine.

When pressed to it, one makes compensations. I came to love winter, when I could wrap up the disfigured lower half of my face in a scarf: I could speak to people and they would have no idea to whom and to what they were really speaking. I developed the bad habits of letting my long hair hang in my face and of always covering my chin and mouth with my hand, hoping it might be mistaken as a thoughtful, accidental gesture. I also became interested in horses and got a job at a run-down local stable. Having those horses to go to each day after school saved my life; I spent all of my time either with them or thinking abut them. Completely and utterly repressed by the time I was sixteen, I was convinced that I would never want a boyfriend, not ever, and wasn't it convenient for me, even a blessing, that none would ever want me. I told myself I was free to concentrate on the "true reality" of life, whatever that was. My sister and her friends put on blue eye shadow, blow-dried their hair, and spent interminable hours in the local mall, and I looked down on them for this, knew they were misleading themselves and being overly occupied with the "mere surface" of living. I'd had thoughts like this when I was younger, ten or twelve, but now my philosophy was haunted by desires so frightening I was unable even to admit they existed.

Throughout all of this, I was undergoing reconstructive surgery in an attempt to rebuild my jaw. It started when I was fifteen, two years after chemo ended. I had known for years I would have operations to fix my face, and at night I fantasized about how good my life would finally be then. One day I got a clue that maybe it wouldn't be so easy. An older plastic surgeon explained the process of "pedestals" to me and told me it would take *ten years* to fix my face. Ten years? Why even bother, I thought, I'll be ancient by then. I went to a medical library and looked up the "pedestals" he talked about. There were gruesome pictures of people with grotesque tubes of their own skin growing out of their bodies, tubes of skin that were harvested like some kind of crop and then rearranged, with results that did not look at all normal or acceptable to my eye. But then I met a younger surgeon who was working on a new way of grafting that did not involve pedestals, and I became more hopeful and once again began to await the fixing of my face, the day when I would be whole, content, loved.

Long-term plastic surgery is not like in the movies. There is no one single operation that will change everything, and there is certainly no slow unwrapping of the gauze in order to view the final, remarkable result. There is always swelling, sometimes to a grotesque degree; there are often bruises; and always there are scars. After each operation, too frightened to simply go look in the mirror, I developed an oblique method, with several stages. First, I tried to catch my reflection in an overhead lamp: the roundness of the metal distorted my image just enough to obscure details and give no true sense of size or proportion. Then I slowly worked my way up to looking at the reflection in someone's eyeglasses, and from there I went to walking as briskly as possible by a mirror, glancing only quickly. I repeated this as many times as it would take me, passing the mirror slightly more slowly each time until finally I was able to stand still and confront myself.

The theory behind most reconstructive surgery is to take large chunks of muscle, skin, and bone and slap them into the roughly appropriate place, then slowly begin to carve this mess into some sort of shape. It involves long, major operations, countless lesser ones, a lot of pain, and many, many years. And also, it does not always work. With my young surgeon in New York, who with each passing year was becoming not so young, I had two or three soft-tissue grafts, two skin grafts, a bone graft, and some dozen other operations to "revise" my face, yet when I left graduate school at the age of twenty-five I was still more or less in the same position I had started in: a deep hole in the right side of my face and a rapidly shrinking left side and chin, a result of the radiation I'd had as a child and the stress placed on the bone by the other operations. I was caught in a cycle of having a big operation, one that would force me to look monstrous from the swelling for many months, then having the subsequent revision operations that improved my looks tremendously, and then slowly, over the period of a few months or a year, watching the graft resorb back into my body, slowly shrinking down and leaving me with nothing but the scarred donor site the graft had originally come from.

It wasn't until I was in college that I finally allowed that maybe, just maybe, it might be nice to have a boyfriend. I went to a small, liberal, predominantly female school and suddenly, after years of alienation in high school, discovered that there were other people I could enjoy talking to who thought me intelligent and talented. I was, however, still operating on the assumption that no one, not ever, would be physically attracted to me, and in a curious way this shaped my personality. I became forthright and honest in the way that only the truly self-confident are, who do not expect to be rejected, and in the way of those like me, who do not even dare to ask acceptance from others and therefore expect no rejection. I had come to know myself as a person, but I would be in graduate school before I was literally, physically able to use my name and the word "woman" in the same sentence.

Now my friends repeated for me endlessly that most of it was in my mind, that, granted, I did not look like everyone else, but that didn't mean I looked bad. I am sure now that they were right some of the time. But with the constant surgery I was in a perpetual state of transfiguration. I rarely looked the same for more than six months at a time. So ashamed of my face, I was unable even to admit that this constant change affected me; I told everyone who wanted to know that it was only what was inside that mattered, that I had "grown used to" the surgery, that none of it bothered me at all. Just as I had done in childhood, I pretended nothing was wrong, and this was constantly mistaken by others for bravery. I spent a great deal of time looking in the mirror in private, positioning my head to show off my eyes and nose, which were not only normal but quite pretty, as my friends told me often. But I could not bring myself to see them for more than a moment: I looked in the mirror and saw not the normal upper half of my face but only the disfigured lower half.

People still teased me. Not daily, as when I was younger, but in ways that caused me more pain than ever before. Children stared at me, and I learned to cross the street to avoid them; this bothered me, but not as much as the insults I got from men. Their taunts came at me not because I was disfigured but because I was a disfigured *woman*. They came from boys, sometimes men, and almost always from a group of them. I had long, blond hair, and I also had a thin figure. Sometimes, from a distance, men would see a thin blond and whistle, something I dreaded more than anything else because I knew that as they got closer, their tune, so to speak, would inevitably change; they would stare openly or, worse, turn away quickly in shame or repulsion. I decided to cut my hair to avoid any misconception that anyone, however briefly, might have about my being attractive. Only two or three times have I ever been teased by a single person, and I can think of only one time when I was ever teased by a woman. Had I been a man, would I have had to walk down the street while a group of young women followed and denigrated my sexual worth?

Not surprisingly, then, I viewed sex as my salvation. I was sure that if only I could get someone to sleep with me, it would mean I wasn't ugly, that I was attractive, even lovable. This line of reasoning led me into the beds of several manipulative men who liked themselves even less than they liked me, and I in turn left each short-term affair hating myself, obscenely sure that if only I had been prettier it would have worked—he would have loved me and it would have been like those other love affairs that I was certain "normal" women had all the time. Gradually, I became unable to say "I'm depressed" but could say only "I'm ugly," because the two had become inextricably linked in my mind. Into that universal lie, that sad equation of "if only . . ." that we are all prey to, I was sure that if only I had a normal face, then I would be happy.

The new surgeon in Scotland, Oliver Fenton, recommended that I undergo a procedure involving something called a tissue expander, followed by a bone graft. A tissue expander is a small balloon placed under the skin and then slowly blown up over the course of several months, the object being to stretch out the skin and create room and cover for the new bone. It's a bizarre, nightmarish thing to do to your face, yet I was hopeful about the end results and I was also able to spend the three months that the expansion took in the hospital. I've always felt safe in hospitals: they're the one place I feel free from the need to explain the way I look. For this reason the first tissue expander was bearable—just—and the bone graft that followed it was a success; it did not melt away like the previous ones.

The surgical stress this put upon what remained of my original jaw instigated the deterioration of that bone, however, and it became unhappily apparent that I was going to need the same operation I'd just had on the right side done to the left. I remember my surgeon telling me this at an outpatient clinic. I had planned to be traveling down to London that same night on an overnight train, and I barely made it to the station on time, such a fumbling state of despair was I in.

I could not imagine going through it *again,* and just as I had done all my life, I searched and searched through my intellect for a way to make it okay, make it bearable, for a way to *do* it. I lay awake all night on that train, feeling the tracks slip beneath me with an odd eroticism, when I remembered an afternoon from my three months in the hospital. Boredom was a big problem those long afternoons, the days marked by meals and television programs. Waiting for the afternoon tea to come, wondering desperately how I could make time pass, it had suddenly occurred to me that I didn't have to make time pass, that it would do it of its own accord, that I simply had to relax and take no action. Lying on the train, remembering that, I realized I had no obligation to improve my situation, that I didn't have to explain or understand it, that I could just simply let it happen. By the time the train pulled into King's Cross station, I felt able to bear it again, not entirely sure what other choice I had.

But there was an element I didn't yet know about. When I returned to Scotland to set up a date to have the tissue expander inserted, I was told quite casually that I'd be in the hospital only three or four days. Wasn't I going to spend the whole expansion time in the hospital? I asked in a whisper. What's the point of that? came the answer. You can just come in every day to the outpatient ward to have it expanded. Horrified by this, I was speechless. I would have to live and move about in the outside world with a giant balloon inside the tissue of my face? I can't remember what I did for the next few days before I went into the hospital, but I vaguely recall that these days involved a great deal of drinking alone in bars and at home.

I had the operation and went home at the end of the week. The only things that gave me any comfort during the months I lived with my tissue expander were my writing and Franz Kafka. I started a novel and completely absorbed myself in it, writing for hours each day. The only way I could walk down the street, could stand the stares I received, was to think to myself, "I'll bet none of them are writing a novel." It was that strange, old, familiar form of egomania, directly related to my dismissive, conceited thoughts during adolescence. As for Kafka, who had always been one of my favorite writers, he helped me in that I felt permission to feel alienated, and to have that alienation be okay, bearable, noble even. In the same way that imagining I lived in Cambodia helped me as a child, I walked the streets of my dark little Scottish city by the sea and knew without doubt that I was living in a story Kafka would have been proud to write.

The one good thing about a tissue expander is that you look so bad with it that no matter what you look like once it's finally removed, your face has to look better. I had my bone graft and my fifth soft-tissue graft and, yes, even I had to admit I looked better. But I didn't look like me. Something was wrong: Was *this* the face I had waited through eighteen years and almost thirty operations for? I somehow just couldn't make what I saw in the mirror correspond to the person I thought I was. It wasn't only that I continued to feel ugly; I simply could not conceive of the image as belonging to me. My own image was the image of a stranger, and rather than try to understand this, I simply stopped looking in the mirror. I perfected the technique of brushing my teeth without a mirror, grew my hair in such a way that it would require only a quick, simple brush, and wore clothes that were simply and easily put on, no complex layers or lines that might require even the most minor of visual adjustments.

On one level I understood that the image of my face was merely that, an image, a surface that was not directly related to any true, deep definition of the self. But I also knew that it is only through appearances that we experience and make decisions about the everyday world, and I was not always able to gather the strength to prefer the deeper world to the shallower one. I looked for ways to find a bridge that would allow me access to both, rather than riding out the constant swings between peace and anguish. The only direction I had to go in to achieve this was to strive for a state of awareness and self-honesty that sometimes, to this day, rewards me. I have found, I believe, that our lives are dominated, though it is not always so clearly translatable, by the question, "How do I look?" Take all the many nouns in our lives—car, house, job, family, love, friends—and substitute the personal pronoun "I." It is not that we are all so self-obsessed; it is that all things eventually relate back to ourselves, and it is through our own sense of how we appear to the world that we chart our lives, that we navigate our personalities, which would otherwise be adrift in the ocean of *other* people's obsessions.

One evening toward the end of my year-long separation from the mirror, I was sitting in a café talking to someone—an attractive man, as it happened—and we were having a lovely, engaging conversation. For some reason I suddenly wondered what I looked like to him. What was he *actually* seeing when he saw me? So many times I've asked this of myself, and always the answer is this: a warm, smart woman, yes, but an unattractive one. I sat there in the café and asked myself this old question, and startlingly, for the first time in my life, I had no answer readily prepared. I had not looked in a mirror for so long that I quite simply had no clue as to what I looked like. I studied the man as he spoke; my entire life I had seen my ugliness reflected back to me. But now, as reluctant as I was to admit it, the only implication in my companion's behavior was positive.

And then, that evening in that café, I experienced a moment of the freedom I'd been practicing for behind my Halloween mask all those years ago. But whereas as a child I expected my liberation to come as a result of gaining something, a new face, it came to me now as a result of shedding something, of shedding my image. I once thought that truth was eternal, that when you understood something it was with you forever. I know now that this isn't so, that most truths are inherently unretainable, that we have to work hard all our lives to remember the most basic things. Society is no help; it tells us again and again that we can most be ourselves by looking like someone else, leaving our own faces behind to turn into ghosts that will inevitably resent and haunt us. It is no mistake that in movies and literature the dead sometimes know they are dead only after they can no longer see themselves in the mirror; and as I sat there feeling the warmth of the cup against my palm, this small observation seemed like a great revelation to me. I wanted to tell the man I was with about it, but he was involved in his own topic and I did not want to interrupt him, so instead I looked with curiosity toward the window behind him, its night-darkened glass reflecting the whole café, to see if I could, now, recognize myself.

diane ackerman

Diane Ackerman's odyssey into the heart and soul of vanilla is as soothing—and healing—as any medicinal remedy for stress or prescription for blissful enjoyment. Ackerman's effectiveness is anchored in her ability to entice the reader into sharing a passion for the subjects that intrigue her.

in praise of vanilla

Craving vanilla, I start the bathwater gushing and unscrew the lid of a heavy glass jar of Ann Steeger of Paris's Bain Creme, *senteur vanille*. A wallop of potent vanilla hits my nose as I reach into the lotion, let it seep through my fingers, and carry a handful to the faucet. Fragrant bubbles fill the tub. A large bar of vanilla bath soap sitting in an antique porcelain dish, acts as an aromatic beacon. While I steep in waves of vanilla, a friend brings me a vanilla cream seltzer, followed by a custard made with vanilla beans that have come all the way from Madagascar. Brown flecks float through the creamy yellow curds. Though I could have chosen beans from the Seychelles, Tahiti, Polynesia, Uganda, Mexico, the Tonga Islands, Java, Indonesia, the Comoro Islands, and other places, I like the long, sensuous shape of the Madagascar vanilla bean, and its dark, rich pliable coat, which looks like carefully combed tresses or the pelt of a small aquatic animal. Some connoisseurs prefer the shorter Tahitian bean, which is fatter and moister (even though it has less vanillin and the moistness is only water, not flavorful oils), or the smoky flavor of beans from Java (wood fires do some of the curing), or the maltier flavor of those from the Comoros.

Most of the world's real vanilla comes from the islands in the Indian Ocean (Madagascar, Reunion, Comoros), which produce a thousand tons of vanilla beans every year. But we rarely taste the real thing. The vanilla flavoring we find in most of our ice creams, cakes, yogurts, and other foods, as well as in shampoos and perfumes, is an artificial flavor created in laboratories and mixed with alcohol and other ingredients. Marshall McLuhan once warned that we were drifting so far away from the real taste of life that we had begun to *prefer* artificiality and were becoming content with eating the menu descriptions rather than the food. Most people have used the medicinal-smelling artificial vanilla flavoring for so long that they have no idea what real vanilla extract tastes and smells like. Real vanilla, with its complex veils of aroma and juggling flavors, makes the synthetic seem a poor parody. Vanillin isn't the only flavor in genuine vanilla, but it's the only one synthetically produced (originally from clove oil, coal tar, and other unlikely substances, but now mainly from the sulfite by-products of paper manufacturing). Indeed, the world's largest producer of synthetic vanillin is the Ontario Paper Company! Real vanilla varies along a spectrum from sweet and dusty to damp and loamlike, depending on the variety of the bean, its freshness, its home country, how and for how long it was cured and in what temper of sun.

When a vanilla bean lies like a Hindu rope on the counter, or sits in a cup of coffee, its aroma gives the room a kind of stature, the smell of an exotic crossroads where outlandish foods aren't the only mysteries. In Istanbul in the 1970s, my mother and I once ate Turkish pastries redolent with vanilla, glazed in caramel sugar with delicate filaments of syrup on top. It was only later that day, when we strolled through the bazaar with two handsome university students my mother had bumped into, that we realized what we had eaten with such relish. On a long brass platter sat the kind of pastries we had eaten, buzzed over by hundreds of sugar-delirious bees, whose feet had gotten stuck in the syrup; desperately, one by one, they flew away, leaving their legs behind. "Bee legs!" my mother had screamed, as her face curdled. "We ate *bee legs!*" Our companions spoke little English and we spoke no Turkish, so they probably thought it odd that American women became so excitable in the presence of pastry. They offered to buy us some, which upset my mother even more.

Walk through a kitchen where vanilla beans are basking in a

loud conundrum of smell, and you'll make some savoring murmur without realizing it. The truth about vanilla is that it's as much a smell as a taste. Saturate your nose with glistening, soulful vanilla, and you can *taste* it. It's not like walking through a sweetshop, but more subterranean and wild. Surely this is the unruly beast itself, the raw vanilla that's clawing your senses. But no. The vanilla beans we treasure aren't delectable the way we find them in the jungle. Of all the foods grown in the world, vanilla requires the most labor: Long, tedious hours of hand tending bring the vanilla orchids to fruit and then the fruit to luciousness. Vanilla comes from the string-bean-like pod of a climbing orchid, whose greenish-white flowers bloom briefly and are without fragrance. Since the blossoms last only one day, they must be hand-pollinated exactly on schedule. The beams mature six weeks after fertilization, but cannot be picked for some months longer. When a bean turns perfectly ripe, the pickers plunge it into boiling water to stop the ripening; they dry and process it, using blankets, ovens, racks, and sweating boxes; and slowly cure it in the sun for six to nine months. The glorious scent and taste don't adorn the growing plant. It's only as the beans ferment to wrinkled, crackly brown pods that the white dots of vanillin crystallize mellowly on their outsides and that famous robust aroma starts to saturate the air.

It was in 1518 that Cortes first noticed the Aztecs flavoring their chocolate with ground-up vanilla pods, which they called *tlilxochitl* ("black flower") and prized so highly that Montezuma drank an infusion of it as a royal balm and demanded vanilla beans in tribute from his subjects. The Spaniards called the bean *vainilla* ("small sheath"), from the Latin *vagina*—the beans' elongated shape, with a slit at the top, must have reminded the lonesome Spaniards of what they were missing. There would have been many boisterous jokes about Montezuma stirring his chocolate with a little vagina.* Cortes

*Randy workmen and explorers are responsible for a lot of interesting etymology. Consider the word "gasket," which come from the Old French, *garcette,* a little girl with her hymen still intact.

valued vanilla enough to carry bags of it back to Europe, along with the Aztecs' gold, silver, jewels, and chocolate. A passion for vanilla, especially in combination with chocolate, raged in Europe, where it was prized as an aphrodisiac. Thomas Jefferson's letters include an appeal to a Parisian friend to send him some vanilla beans, for which he had developed a taste during his tenure as the U.S. minister to France, and which he couldn't find in American apothecary shops.

Precious and desirable as vanilla was, no one could figure out how to grow it outside of Mexico. The problem was typical of how fragile all the lush green abandon really is, but no one realized it. Though insects, birds, and bats pollinate most plants in the tropics, the vanilla orchid is pollinated by only one type of bee, the tiny melipone. In 1836, a Belgian figured out the vanilla orchid's secret sex life when he caught sight of the melipone bumbling about its work. Then the French devised a method of hand-pollinating the orchids and started plantations on their Indian Ocean islands, as well as in the East and West Indies. The Dutch carried vanilla to Indonesia, and the British to India.

"Tincture of vanilla" didn't appear in the United States until the 1800s, but when it did, it appealed to the American impatience and aversion to fuss, that sprint through life whose byword is *convenience*. Europeans used the vanilla bean, luxuriating in its textures, tastes, and aromas, but we preferred it reduced and already bottled. By the nineteenth century, demand flourished, vanilla became synthesized, and the world floated on a mantle of cheap flavoring. Vanilla now appears as an ingredient in most baked goods and in many perfumes, cleaning products, and even toys, and has insinuated itself into the cuisine of far-flung peoples, conquering their palates. Only saffron is a more expensive spice.

When I finally emerge from the tub into which I had climbed at the beginning of this discussion, I apply Ann Steeger's vanilla body veil, which smells edible and thick as smoke. Then Jean Laporte's vanilla perfume, vanilla with a bitter sting. The inside of a vanilla bean contains a figlike marrow, and if I were to scrape some out, I could prepare spicy vanilla bisque for dinner, followed by chicken in a vanilla glaze, salad with vanilla vinaigrette, vanilla ice cream with a sauce of chestnuts in vanilla marinade, followed by warm brandy flavored with chopped vanilla pod, and then, in a divine vanilla stupor, seep into bed and fall into a heavy orchidlike sleep.*

*To make real vanilla extract: Split a vanilla bean lengthwise, set in a glass jar, cover with ¾ cup of vodka. Cover and let steep for at least six weeks. As you use the extract, add more vodka; the bean will stay redolent and continue oozing flavor for some time. Add a teaspoon of vanilla extract to French toast batter to transmogrify it into the New Orleans version called "lost bread." Vanilla sugar tastes wonderful in coffee: Split one vanilla bean from top to bottom and cut into pieces; mix with two cups of sugar; cover; let stand for six weeks. The longer the vanilla stands, the more intense the flavor.

raphael campo

Campo is healed—and reaffirmed—by the act of writing. In this narrative, he bares his soul, details intima-
cies with riveting candor. It is the specificity of his
language and his willingness to reveal himself without
alibi and explanation that makes this essay so believ-
able—and acceptable.

dora rewriting freud:
desiring to heal

His erection startled me. At first, it seemed merely to point me out, acknowledging my part in the simple and various human desires present in our encounter—the desire to be loved and to be healed, the desire to be naked before another and thus to be utterly understood and to be wordlessly explained, the desire for a life beyond this one, the desire to represent what is the truth. What could be more natural than that I was there, a witness to another man's ailing body. For a fleeting moment, I too wished to be naked, to be as available to him in his suffering as he had made himself to me. The sheer exclamation of the pleasure in one person's touching the body of another—I have been a doctor long enough to know what joy and power there is in the laying on of hands—must have frightened me, so explicit and insistent it was in this form. Gradually, I let myself become aware of my stethoscope, my white coat, my cold hands in their latex gloves as they all continuously emitted their signals. The entire milieu of my chilly, fluorescently lit office seemed to be warning us both of my very great distance. I watched as if from behind the surveillance camera of my years of medical training as I mutated into an alien space scientist, studying and cataloging a curious lifeform on a forbidding planet. Then I excused myself abruptly, saying in an oddly flat voice that I needed to get more liquid nitrogen to finish burning off the warts. I let the door slam shut loudly, definitively, behind me.

In considering later what had occurred between this patient and me, I found myself revisiting what had drawn me to medicine in the first place. Before I was completely aware of it, I had begun to write feverishly at my cluttered desk, allowing myself to feel the presence of his body again, to touch his fragrant skin—I suddenly recalled his spicy cologne—without the barrier of my rubbery gloves. Whether it was another poem, or a long love letter, or the beginning of this book, I cannot be sure. What I do know is that in the act of writing I encountered again the shocking, empowering energy of a great desire. A desire that I have always known belongs to all of us.

My earliest conscious recollections of disturbances within my own body are those of the minor bumps and bruises whose pain was alleviated by my parents' kisses. Kissing was the most potent and intoxicating of all elixirs. Pure physical contact had the power to cure. My body, before I was capable of truly hurting myself, could be reconstituted with my mother's moist breath in my ear as she sang me a comforting song. The pleasures I felt, more intelligible to the child's mind than my parents likely suspected, are in great part what led me later in life to the healing arts. I desired to be made well in their eyes, to be acceptable, to be beautiful, to be kissed. My desiring of my parents had a good deal of its expression in the ritual of the tearfully extended, oftentimes exaggerated "boo-boo," presented for their fastidious attention. To be well meant to be well loved.

Music and magic, and particularly their expression and absorption in the physical body, were the primary modes of healing recoverable in the bits and shreds of Cuban culture that I encountered as a child. My grandmother's dark bedroom, its windows covered by thick red velvet draperies as if to keep out the weak winter light and the images of scrawny trees, seemed a shrine dedicated to the various saints before whom she lit candles as offerings. I would hear her praying or singing quietly in Spanish, believing perhaps that she was restoring health to an infirm relative back in Cuba whom she would never see again. Though I could not understand most of what she said, I let my heart be carried by her evident hope that her words could reach across the oceans. In her songs, my mind was transported all the way from sickly Elizabeth, New Jersey, and its bleak refineries and landfills, to the verdant, lush Cuban countryside I imagined was her real home. Healing had a voice and seemed rooted in a most potent physical longing, a longing to be with the ones you loved. Later in childhood, my family's Venezuelan maid Bonifacia would make special potions from tropical juices and other secret ingredients for me and my brothers. Some potions caused laughter; others could restore friendship or ease the pain of a lost pet. I still believe in the inherent magical properties of her concoctions, just as I understand the placebo effect: she too taught me that healing is a consequence in some measure of what the mind desires.

As I grew older, the connections multiplied between doctoring and desire. At around the age of eight, my cousins, friends, and I began "playing doctor." This enactment of adulthood was all the permission we needed to examine our own and each other's genitals freely and without shame. Though the myriad implications of our sexual acts were not yet within the realms of our conscious imaginations, we did guess capably at what might fit where. Fingers to vagina, penis to anus, mouth to nipple, each combination we employed shedding more light on the body's functions and sources of pleasure. Listening to the heart, ear pressed to the bare chest of a playmate, was the opening of a vast interior world. What did another person contain? The ingredients listed in our nursery rhymes—sugar, snails, spice, and puppy dog tails—seemed unlikely, even impossible. Whatever really constituted a person, the essence of the body felt very, very good.

At around the same time, I began to learn to fear what another's heart might contain. I recall the particular experience of playing doctor with my best friend, and his mother discovering us with our pants down in a hall closet, flashlights pointed at each other's dicks. She screamed and angrily beat my friend before my eyes with one of the flashlights—the very instrument of our mutual and brief enlightenment. Our happy curiosity and arousal were suddenly transformed and redefined as shameful in a moment's judgment. Our queerness was apparent, revolting, and indisputable. The bandages in which we wrapped my friend afterward were blindingly white, the blood stains that soaked through them were grotesquely real, the iodine made him wince and cry visible tears. The body now bore the imprint of pain, bruises and welts written upon the skin like a language all too terribly familiar. Healing also had its origins in injury and insult, and so was a potentially painful process, not a uniformly pleasurable one. Desire had its consequences.

Just as the body could be made legible by violence, I also came to learn that the body itself could write upon the world. It could remake its very form. My own body changed under the influence of puberty's hormonal surge and weight lifting. On the soccer field, my movements became more purposeful and effective, and my approach to the sport took on the quality of narrative, as if through a game a story could be told, a deeper meaning expressed. Hair and muscle sprang up on me, announcing my sex ever more urgently. I walked differently, advertising myself to other teenagers. My penis enlarged and demanded much more of my attention. I grasped it like a megaphone, ready to shout at the top of my lungs at how unimaginably wonderful it felt as I came. A few of my friends and I masturbated together, boastfully comparing the sizes of our dicks but never daring to touch one another.

It is not surprising, then, that it was during adolescence, as my body began to speak its language of desire more boldly to the outside world, that I also began to understand medicine as a "desirable" profession. My parents, dedicated as they were to ensuring their children's security and success, urged me to consider a career as a physician. As a child of immigrants, I imagined that my white coat might make up for, possibly even purify, my nonwhite skin; learning the medical jargon might be the ultimate refutation of any questions about what my first language had been. Meanwhile, medicine was becoming a force in shaping (or in cleaning up) the culture—through government-sponsored public health messages about smoking, exercise, and drugs—that filtered into my consciousness. Dr. Ruth became wildly popular, her strong German accent communicating her scientific detachment and clinical coolness. Gym and sex education classes took on a distinctly wholesome tone, intent on sanitizing our minds and bodies. Stodgy gray-haired physicians who practiced in our upper-middle-class community came to school and gave solemn talks about VD and the evils of smoking pot to assemblies in the gleaming multipurpose room.

I memorized biology homework assignments full of meiosis, gametocytes, zygotes, and stark reproduction: perhaps science could pin down the definition of desire, I thought, with a mixture of hope and terror. In Sunday school lessons I had learned about Adam and Eve, and read Genesis; the biblical Eden in which they dwelled was unfailingly depicted as brightly hygienic, obsessively neat, and monotonously sunny. Their secular counterparts were laden with an equally insidious morality, the suburban white couples with emerald green lawns who were my family's neighbors, who shared our near paradise of flowering trees that bore inedible fruit and of sparkling undrinkable water in chlorinated pools. In science class, alongside their children, I dissected frogs and cats beneath the sterile fluorescent lights, and all our instruments were autoclaved at the end of the day. I remember laying open the reproductive organs; how tidy, glistening, and clean the pickled genitals seemed. The body, I was taught, was the most immaculate of machines.

When a beautiful young woman in my class with long red hair got body lice, a sort of panic ensued in our high school. It was as though a witch had been discovered, and when her parents burned her favorite jeans and black concert T-shirts, and then had her head shaved, our teachers appeared to be relieved and pleased. The message of this group hysteria seemed to be that the purpose of the body was healthful reproduction, and a relentless self-control over its processes and smallest environments was the only business of life. The pathologizing of not only tobacco and alcohol but also of the out-of-control, "dirty," and "addictive" consumption of sexual pleasure and food became the other side of the medical coin.

By my junior year my favorite teacher in high school was Mr. H., a middle-aged man with graying temples and an evident passion for his subject matter. He taught Advanced Placement Biology and was building an electron microscope himself. He was not exactly handsome; I recall other teachers commenting once that he was "smarmy." His hands and his veined arms would become covered in chalk dust as he diagrammed anatomical structures. After school, he dirtied himself with black grease assembling his microscope. When he taught us, he engaged us with his entire formidable body, running frantically up and down the aisles, heaving his chest as he bellowed out questions, coaxing answers out from even the shyest of mouths. His lectures were more invigorating and draining than the calisthenics of gym class. Surely no one failed to notice his tremendous bulging crotch, his tight polyester pants stretched almost painfully over his obvious hard-on. He injected a sexual energy into the classroom to which I was unaccustomed and attracted. We learned insatiably from him. He transfused the lifeblood of his risky enthusiasm into our anemic textbooks.

Mr. H. was never the hygienic physician clad in a spotless white coat who Marcus Welby was portrayed to be. His poorly concealed affair with a female classmate of mine was eventually made public by them both, to the young woman's parents and to Mr. H.'s wife (from whom we all later learned he had been long separated). Mr. H. was asked to resign the next day, despite protests from the students in his classes. The humiliation and dejection in his eyes was apparent as he made his chaste announcement. Science became an ever more frightening arena indeed, where matters of the heart, excepting of course its laborious physiology, were disallowed entirely and, if pursued, led to the sternest of punishments. Passion could and indeed must be regulated, and especially the excited intercourse between teacher and student, scientist and layperson, and by extension, I began to suspect, between the mythic physician and his vulnerable patient.

In this environment I too became enraged and indignant upon reading the increasingly frequent and prurient reports in the media of chemistry teachers molesting their impressionable students, psychiatrists seducing their hypnotized subjects, and dentists fondling their anesthetized patients. A facile self-righteousness arose in me, paralleling my growing awareness of my differentness from those around me. I began imagining myself as the model physician, for whom desire was forbidden and in fact repellent, which served to defend me from my growing and undeniable sexual interest in other men. I thought I could cure myself of my own emerging identities; perhaps drinking too much guava nectar and listening too intently to merengues had made me too obviously Cuban, or masturbating too much had made me gay. I had nearly come full circle in my beliefs. In my fear of what I might become, and in accordance with what I had been taught, I reinterpreted the body as designed for orderly reproduction and not love or pleasure, for harboring low levels of cholesterol and triglycerides, not the rich voice of the soul. My grandmother, my parents, Bonifacia, and my queer playmates disintegrated in the bright glare of my self-examination.

I lost twenty pounds as a premed during my sophomore year of college; the more I desired anything, especially the man who has since become my lover of the past eleven years, the less I permitted myself to eat. At the same time, I exercised obsessively, so that I was utterly exhausted at the end of each day. Though I studied my premedical course materials frantically, I loathed the thought of visiting a doctor for the worsening pain in my left upper abdomen. After a prolonged period of time around midterms, when my increasing intake of Diet Coke and Marlboros precluded that of food—my base appetites were almost completely suppressed—I felt a pain in my left side so sharp that I forced myself to dial Campus Emergency. Minutes later, lying naked except for a flimsy gown on one of the Student Health Services examining-room tables, I had a fantasy that was almost overpowering in its vividness. My attending physician was an older Mr. H., and though his strong physical presence seemed undiminished, his voice and his manner had grown much gentler. When he spoke, the pain ceased. He examined me without stethoscopes, reflex hammers, or electrocardiographic leads. When he rested his head on my chest, I could feel him listening to my heart and lungs, understanding all that I had for so long found impossible to say. He then ran his hands over my body, extracting each gossamer toxin that was a shadow of my form and dissolving it in a pool of sunlight. That is when I realized that he was naked too and that I was not ashamed of my urgent erection. Indeed, I felt a certain inexplicable power.

The door opened unexpectedly, putting a rather abrupt end to my dream. Then there was the clatter of a clipboard on a metal countertop, the cold stethoscope, the clumsy, almost punitive lubricated finger. I was given some intravenous fluid and, upon coming to my senses, was given the diagnosis of a pulled intercostal muscle. Reassurance, it appeared, was the only medicine I needed. I returned to my dorm dumbfounded and feeling more than a bit silly. It was only much later that I realized what had occurred in those few hours when I feared I was dying, even wished that I might die: I had located an intersection between my own mortality and the world around me, which was named desire. I wanted to live and to be loved, and at the same time I yearned to erase myself from the face of the earth. I wanted the morguelike steel and chill of the doctor's office and the warm hands of another upon my body telling me by his touch that I would endure.

Not long after this incident, I made love to my best friend for the first time, confirming what we had known for almost two years. What barrier it was that had been removed by my experience of illness, I could not have articulated then. I can report now, however, the healing I felt in each kiss, each touch, each murmured word. My body belonged to me again, as soon as I had owned its desire. To examine the crossing of this threshold—from bodily illness to mental health, from repressed misanthrope to unabashed queer—I changed my scientific methodology from neurophysiology to prosody, my tools from physics equations to rhyme, my materials from atoms to phonemes. If straight science could not provide the vocabulary I needed, perhaps the mysterious and complex human body could explain itself to me in its own terms.

It is through language, then, that I have found a way to love my patients, to desire them and thus put to work one of the most powerful elements of the therapeutic relationship. Present in my poetry is both the rhythm of my grandmother's praying and the thudding of a flashlight striking flesh. I am healing myself when I write, dancing close to another's body to a favorite Spanish song, allowing my mouth to find another man's mouth, because writing itself is the meeting of two expressive surfaces, that of the mind and that of the page. I can press my ear to my patients' chests in each lyric and lie down for the long night beside them in each narrative. The pleasure in touching their skin I experience again in the pleasure my hand creates as it brushes against the smooth page. The love I feel for them is in the beating iambic heart of my lyrics.

The image of the page as yet unwritten upon conjures up powerfully an image of my patient Mary, smoothly bald and pale white from chemotherapy. On the bone marrow transplant unit, because most patients stay for such long periods of time, hospital rooms are transformed even more undeniably into their bedrooms. Each morning during my rounds I would visit Mary in hers. Our encounters were always preceded by my ritualistic hand washing, obeying the strict rules to prevent infection, as the bone marrow ablation therapy she had undergone left her devoid of the cells responsible for immune function. She could not have been more naked, more available and accessible to others, more beautifully free. As I let the warm water run over my hands, I would begin to forget that the soap I was using was bactericidal, as the killing of even the smallest of organisms seemed to have no place in our growing intimacy. I imagined at times that I was visiting a secret love, so much urgency did I feel in her desire to live. We spoke in hushed tones, hardly a word about the progress of her cell counts, more and more about silly, temporary things like our favorite Chinese restaurants, how much we each owed in parking tickets, the nurse's new butch haircut. On and on, like teenagers in a booth at a soda fountain. When I'd leave, I'd fear during the long hours I was away from her that I might never see her again. When I'd cry, she'd tell me to shut up. Wondering whether she felt the same way I did, I'd feel my heart quicken at the slightest intercourse: my ungainly otoscope whispering light into her ears, my slinky stethoscope hearing her heart's demand to live, my stiff penlight prompting the inexplicably delicious constriction of her pupils.

Many doctors must fall in love with their patients, though far, far fewer would likely dare admit it. What else were we to do, one of us dying less quickly than the other, the other less capable of preventing death than the first. So we loved each other in the ways that we could. We listened to each other attentively and held hands. I write about her now, and she is alive. Constrained as we were by our respective worldly roles, as doctor and patient, gay Latino man and straight white woman, still we found the space to make a very particular kind of love—a love that concerned itself less with gender than with transcendence. Highly erotic and deeply pleasuring without our ever having slept together, as commonplace and yet unexpected as life crossing over to death, as immortal as each retelling or the act of writing. Both Mary and I left our loving friendship healthier, I think, closer to being cured. She waved to me as she left the hospital, still bald, still beautiful, but more full of life, the life we shared.

However, I remain fearful for the future of this sort of honesty. The so-called personal lives of physicians and patients—as if the organs of emotion could be so carefully dissected in such an acute relationship—are already the subject of a scrutiny that seeks to eradicate the possibility of human connections. One need look no further than the cover of a major newsmagazine that appeared not too long ago to see the face of a physician so many now fear; ironically, though it was an image meant to sensationalize, it is to me a face as exquisite in its beauty as those of so many of my patients. The story was about a possibly homosexual dentist with AIDS who allegedly infected several of his patients with the virus and died leaving behind a furor: *How did he give it to them,* the text of the article insistently asks.

I am certain that the hysteria around the issues of doctors with AIDS reflects at least in part the deep anxieties that come with recognizing the desire inherent in the patient-doctor relationship. Such fears remain pervasive in the culture at large, specifically with regard to the queerness inherent in a profession that in its practice crosses so many boundaries. Suddenly every lurking suspicion could be true, and each resentment is justified. The bespectacled, nerdy older man sticking his colonoscope up your ass actually *likes* it; worse yet, so might you. The image of sick physician as queer parallels the equation of AIDS = gay man. So it is not surprising that the same old sanitizing tactics have once again become implemented, with rules having been laid down as to which procedures are "safe" for HIV-positive physicians to perform and which are not—without a single shred of scientific evidence to suggest that the virus could even be transmitted through the contact such guidelines seek to limit.

People with AIDS, of course, were the subject of aggressive attempts at quarantine long before the public at large began to mistrust its physicians. Doctors themselves, it seems, could all too capably imagine the intimate contact they might have with their patients; the preexisting mechanisms for control present in the profession made it even easier for physicians to insulate themselves from people with AIDS under their care. During medical school I often overheard interns, residents, and attending physicians trying to guess which patients were most likely to give them AIDS through some vividly imagined mishap: the effeminate patient who squeals and jerks his arm away abruptly during a blood draw and thereby causes a needlestick, the normal-appearing hemophiliac who undergoes emergency surgery for appendicitis, the drug addict who vomits forcefully into the face of the rescuer performing chest compressions during an overdose-related cardiac arrest. In some cases, those patients known to have AIDS would receive less attentive care because of such fears. To this day, some surgeons outright refuse to operate on patients with AIDS, even on those they only suspect might harbor the virus. Other physicians simply insist on proof of seronegativity before undertaking any invasive procedure.

As a new intern on the wards in San Francisco, I too fell prey to fears of AIDS, each emaciated body I encountered seeming a potential version of me. I saw my own face over and over again in their faces, the dark complexions, the mustaches, the self-deprecation. Incapable as I was then of loving my patients, I hated them instead for reminding me that I was no different, that despite my medical knowledge I was not invincible. My well-rehearsed internalized self-loathing dominated my emotional response to them. I wished that they would hurry up and finish dying, all of them in one fell swoop, and that they would take all the dying there was left in the world with them when they did. In time, my heart was gradually pressed out of me, and I blamed my inability to cry on the long, dehydrating hours I spent in the hospital. Instead of making love with my partner on the nights we shared a bed together, I slept fitfully, inhabiting personalized nightmares about AIDS.

In some ways, I know I have been dying of AIDS since the moment I first learned about the virus. Each smooth tube of blood I draw seems to come from my own scarred and indurated veins, each death note I have dictated has my name and signature at the bottom of the page. Any disease that could erase from the world the bodies of so many people like me, people with whom I had not even had the chance to form the bonds of community, would seem necessarily to take with it small parts of my anatomy; AIDS has cut off the part of my tongue that once made it easy for me to sing, it has laser-ablated my seminal vesicles, it has occluded the blood flow to the area of my visual cortex capable of plainly seeing joy. What I had not been doing during those first few months of internship was trying to love despite the virus, or because of the virus. My healing powers, rudimentary as they were then, were hindered by a superficial wish to know death purely and simply as an enemy.

When I met Aurora, she changed everything. At first, she did not speak at all, except with her huge, moist eyes. I had admitted her to the hospital at 2:00 A.M. one grueling on-call night, with the emergency room diagnosis of "AIDS failure to thrive." (It was not until two weeks later that Aurora told me she was dying of love, of too much love; cynically, I assumed she was referring to her own licentiousness.) Aurora was a preoperative male-to-female transsexual, according to some of my colleagues; to others, she was a freak. On our formal rounds at her bedside the next morning my jittery and bumbling attending physician wondered with a nervous laugh what "it" had between "its" legs. Aurora just stared at him with her incredible eyes. I had written the order that she be placed in isolation because her chest X ray was suspicious for tuberculosis. "Consumption," she would murmur to me later, "yes, I believe I am being consumed by my having loved too deeply." I was too busy to notice then the campy melodrama in her tone of voice; I could barely breathe through my protective fiberglass-mesh mask and thought only of getting out of her room as soon as possible.

One day she began to flirt with me. "I know you're in there," she purred into my ear one morning as I mechanically examined her. I paused only briefly before I plugged my ears with my stethoscope with the intention of listening to her heart sounds. Without saying anything, I raised her hospital gown up to her nipples, this time noticing the fullness of her breasts, the rich chocolate color of her nipples, the deep grooves between her delicate ribs. "Do you think I am beautiful?" She brought a crimson silk scarf up to her eyes and peered seductively over it at me. Her eyes were made up in three shades of green, the eyeliner and eyeshadow thickly applied. I had seen her at her mirror only once, hands trembling slightly, as she applied her cosmetics. At that moment I had thought her beautiful, not at all pathetic or threatening or "failing to thrive." She seemed hopeful and human, full of the love she kept so rapturously spilling out to those around her. But I was too busy to give much thought to what I had felt; my job was not to feel but to palpate. Not to love but to diagnose.

During the course of about eight weeks, Aurora gradually deteriorated despite the intravenous fluids and antibiotics. Her cough became more insistent, as though it were finally winning a long, drawn-out argument. She appeared less frequently in her flowing emerald green kimono and stopped putting on her eye makeup. She gossiped less about the other patients and no longer held court in the patient lounge, where she had often been seen pointing out the cute male passersby with her nail file as she manicured herself. I pretended not to see her; I still listened only to her heart sounds and not to her heart. "You know you're gonna be mine," she sang out to me on another day in her naughtiest Spanish Harlem accent, parodying one of the day's popular dance club songs. I rolled my eyes as I left her room. I never said more than a few words to her on my visits. I busied myself instead with collecting the data of her decline: the falling weight, the diminishing oxygen saturation readings, the recurring fevers. "I'm burning for you, honey," she said with arched eyebrows by way of good-bye on the last day she spoke. Again I said nothing.

Expecting her usual chatter more than I ever could have admitted, I strode into her room the next morning without knocking, as was my habit. No salacious remark greeted me, however, no invitation to sit close to her on her bed, no perfume. The silence registered. She seemed to be lying sideways in her bed, with her face half buried in a pillow. The room's curtains had not been drawn open; she remained motionless as I jolted them apart, flooding the bed with sunlight. I glowered impatiently at her from the bedside; still, she did not move. When I rolled her over, seeing her face stripped of all her glittery makeup, expressing not recognition but a deeply subterraneous pain, a primitive and wordless agony, finally I was moved. As I groped for her, finding her body half paralyzed and oddly limp and angular like a bird that has flown into a window-pane, I began to feel broken myself. I was witnessing the loss of love from the world. Finally in its absence I was hearing her voice, and when I frantically listened to her heart and to her lungs for the first and last time I heard the love in them. I heard my own stifled desire surface for air in my long sobs.

Aurora died later that day, and when she died she left behind an element of herself in me. I find her voice in mine, like a lover's fingers running through my hair; my voice sounds warmer, more comfortable to me now. I discover her hands on my own body when I examine a person with cancer, or AIDS, searching for the same familiar human landmarks that bespeak physical longing and intimacy. Her glorious eyes return to me when I finally see someone for the first time, or when my own bring forth tears. Her friendship and her love of life return to the world in these words, in the poems I write that I hope might ascend to reach her in whatever realm she may now exist. Instead of giving me AIDS as I had so irrationally feared, she gave me hope.

Science failed to understand her, though it altered her body. Medicine did not love her, though it penetrated her with needles and X rays. Only the act of writing can find her now, because it is the same journey she has made, from the imagined to the actual, from the transitory to the persistent. From the unspoken to this physical and loving lament.

c. k. williams

These are the beginning and the ending pages of C. K. Williams's memoir, *Misgivings*, published in 2000, the year in which Williams won the Pulitzer Prize for poetry. They capture Williams saying good-bye to his father and reaffirming the war and peace that most men endure through the awesome and unrelenting experience of rebellion and a state of maturity, which is only sporadically achieved. At this moment, Williams is sadly triumphant.

misgivings

My father dead, I come into the room where he lies and I say aloud, immediately concerned that he might still be able to hear me, *What a war we had!* I say it to my father's body, still propped up on its pillows, before the men from the funeral home arrive to put him into their horrid zippered green bag to take him away, before his night table is cleared of the empty bottles of pills he wolfed down when he'd finally been allowed to end the indignity of his suffering, and had found the means to do it. Before my mother comes in to lie down beside him.

When my mother dies, I'll say to her, as unexpectedly, knowing as little that I'm going to, "I love you." But to my father, again now, my voice, as though of its own accord, blurts, *What a war!* And I wonder again why I'd say that. It's been years since my father and I raged at each other the way we once did, violently, rancorously, seeming to loathe, despise, detest one another. Years since we'd learned, perhaps from each other, perhaps each in our struggles with ourselves, that conflict didn't have to be as it had been for so long the routine state of affairs between us.

And yet it was "war" that came out of me now, spontaneously, mindlessly, with such velocity I couldn't have stopped it no matter what, but, still, I don't understand why it's this I'd want to say to my father at the outset of his death. As though memory were as wayward and fractious as dream, as indifferent to emotional reasoning, as resistant to bringing forth meanings or truths, verifications that might accord with any reasonable system of values. As though memory had its own procedures of belief and purpose that exist outside of and beyond our vision of our lives.

With my mother, as I remember again now speaking to her in her death, my memory, capricious as ever, brings her to me on the shore of a lake, in a bathing suit. I'm very young—I don't even have a brother or sister yet. My mother is sitting beside me speaking to my father. Bathing suits are made of wool then, even mine, and I'm acutely aware of how rough the fabric must be to my mother's sensitive skin; its abrasiveness is a violation, a desecration: I try to stroke the skin under the straps on her back. My mother smiles at me. My father smiles, too. In the water later, in the shallows, I teach myself to walk on my hands with my body afloat behind me. "Look, I'm swimming!" I cry out in pride to my mother, who, in my memory, breaking off what she was saying then to my father, smiles at me again.

And yet that other spurt of speech from the past, to my father lying before me, as though we'd never effected our unspoken reconciliation, as though we'd never embraced, never, after our decades of combat, held one another, our cheeks touching, our chests for a moment pressed together—to my father come words that seem to contain an eruption of still painful feelings, though I know those feelings have been transformed, transfigured: peace for rage, affection for frustration, devotion and compassion for misunderstanding.

The first time my father and I kissed each other as adults, the first time we managed to move across and through our old enmities, across and through our thousand reservations, our thousand hesitations; the first time we stood that way together, arms around each other, we seemed to me to be uncannily high from the earth: it was as though I were a child again, suddenly stretched to my father's height as I held him, gazing dizzily down in disbelief at the world far beneath us. My mother was there, watching, saying nothing, taken—surely at least at that moment—with relief for us all, yet too caught in her own timidities and her own travails to dare speak it aloud.

. . .

This was the room in which my father would die. For me now, anything that ever happened in that room can seem to have already present in it those two events: my mother saying what she did to my father, and his death, the death he would will for himself in that same bed; his death rests off to one side, silent, patient, so that my father as my mother speaks to him seems to be lying alongside himself, and the likelihood of his re-plying seems as slight as if my mother were speaking to that future ghost.

I don't really know if her words hurt him, and yet they hurt me, even now. Whenever they come to mind, they arrive with a shock, of shame, of remorse, as though I had to feel for my father what he was incapable of feeling, or of knowing he was feeling. I can still sense, too, as though I were there with them, how the tiny corner of the night their bedroom contained goes utterly still with my mother's waiting for my father to re-ply or not reply, and with his deciding whether he will or won't. Of not deciding: it would have to have been something so deep within him that replied that there couldn't have been any actual decision on his part; any-thing he said would have had to have come out of him spontaneously, without his thinking it first, and he would immediately have had to make clear to both my mother and himself that there was no surrender or sub-mission, even a surrender to whatever in himself had caused him to speak, to be inferred from his response. Submission was an act, a phenomenon, it would have been unthinkable for him to let anyone, even himself, in-flict upon him. An upsurging, then, perhaps of a connection long forgot-ten, long ago put aside so it wouldn't interfere with his crucial interchanges with himself, with the reality he'd shaped to contain those interchanges.

Meanwhile, he still hasn't spoken. I can tell even from here how much he would have wanted to be asleep by then; how much he wishes to be left alone. Can he ever be alone again with her there waiting beside him, having said that? Could he bring himself to ask her to explain, or elaborate on what she'd said? "You used to be such a nice man." Cer-tainly it would have needed explication. Certainly he must have been abashed at having his life so compressed, condensed into what was, after all, considering how circumspect my mother normally was with him, a devastating accusation. Yet I can't find in my memory any evidence to show that what she said changed in any way how he acted during those years. I can't imagine either any reply he might have made to her. There's only the silence, and, for me, that image of his death waiting beside him, already beginning to absorb him.

When I touch my father after his death, when I close his eyes, stroke his face, something shudders in my chest, I reel within myself for a moment, all the muscles of my own face seem to harden, I can think of nothing more to say to him than I've already choked out about our war, though I know there's much I would say if I could. Then it occurs to me that this silence, half-mind, half-body, that's taken me is grief, and I feel that perhaps I'm honoring my father in the one currency that would still have value to him, my anguish for him, my mourning not for having lost him, for he's still here in my emotions and still before me in his flesh, but because I've lost that aspect of him, his existence, the sheer fact of his being, all I'd always kept with me as I blundered through my life.

To my mother I say, "I love you," to my father I speak of war; yet aren't both declarations after all of attachment and allegiance?

My father's glasses are off. Except when he was young, and would take them off for his picture to be taken, he always wore them and always seemed to me unlike himself without them. When I was a child and he'd pretend he was going to wrestle with me, crush me, he'd take his glasses off first, and even before he went into his dance of menace he was already unrecognizable and forbidding. Now, though, without them he seems more himself than he's ever been, even during those last days when he knew he was going and had fiercely reaffirmed his proprietary rights over himself.

I wonder again whether my father would have heard me say

what I said, the way my mother, far, far away in her coma, may have heard my aunt. Would he have understood me and realized why what came to me were words of a recognition neither of us had ever spoken?

Forgiveness is such an elusive act. Why, when we're at last prepared to relinquish our estrangements, when we've all but forgotten the grounds for our disapprobation and are ready at last to speak of the incomprehension that surged though us unsaid, does there seem nothing to be said, and at the end, nothing to forgive? We seem suddenly to have neither the need nor the right to forgive; the very concept of forgiveness can feel repellent and debasing.

And why, too, once having realized and enacted our forgiveness as well as we can, do we at once seem forgiven ourselves, so that sometimes we can mistrust in ourselves our reasons for having forgiven: might our being shriven of blame ourselves be all we really were after? But perhaps forgiveness is a process more than an emotion, perhaps it's meant to make us discover those other conditions within ourselves, love, belief in love, to which forgiveness itself is incidental: perhaps forgiveness once accomplished becomes a condition of existence, a reality as ineluctable as our physical and mental being.

My father and I are silent now. The silence between parent and child, the whir through us of old emotions, the tangled chords of our misunderstandings, the chaotic scraps of never pronounced phrases of explanation and intention: I feel nothing of that.

In the days and weeks and months after my father dies, I'll dream about him often, more than I'd have thought. My mother, when she dies, will take a long time to come to my dreams; when she finally appears it'll be in the most matter-of-fact way, with no fuss at all; she often seems to be smiling at me out of my dream.

But in the first dreams I have of my father, he doesn't seem to know quite where he is; I can sense a lack of assurance in him, a diffidence: he doesn't seem unhappy, but he's terribly uncertain. Often he seems to want to say something to me, but he never can state whatever it is clearly enough for me to understand. As time passes, I have dreams in which he begins to seem alert, content, self-possessed; he's always very involved in what's going on in the dream: when there's a task to be performed, he helps me with it, always in a very unobtrusive way. Then come dreams in which he seems utterly at peace with himself; he moves easily into and through dreams, and comes and goes from them calmly, and his being in a dream and his departure from it are both so unpretentious and guileless that I'm comforted, and released, I'm not sure why, from an apprehension of my own, perhaps from my abiding desire to be other than I am. And that feeling of acceptance stays with me even when I wake; sometimes I think it might be the last gift my father bestowed on me.

Now, waiting next to his body, perhaps I have a premonition of that gift; perhaps I sense that the resignation and serenity of the time before my father's dying has passed on to me, although I don't know yet how all of it will be manifested in me, or when.

What I do now is lift my father's arm, the one that hadn't been broken: it weighs so much, feels so inert, yet it expresses not loss, not incompletion, but a reassuring finality. It makes me feel not as though my father has evaded his real death, escaped his body's destruction and his mind's terror of debility, but as though he's arrived at the state of being he'd set out for from the beginning. I think that perhaps his will has conquered his complexities at last, and his death has brought a fruition he'd never imagined to his will.

I hear my mother in the other room as the rest of the family tries to comfort her. She doesn't really believe yet that my father is dead, though she's been told. Someone has said, "It's over," but she hasn't really understood. Now she comes in, looks for a moment with almost no expression at my father, then lies down next to him, adjacent to but not quite touching him, and her eyes close. I watch them both, my mother and father, I watch myself watching, then I go.

debra spark

To paraphrase Debra Spark's last line, this essay is so real, so vivid, so well executed, so "delicious" . . . the reader will want to cry. Spark moves from past to present, third person to first person, with cinematic brilliance. Her sister and their relationship remain vivid on the page because she is able to employ an array of literary techniques—dialogue, scene, suspense, reflection, action—while representing various and conflicting points of view.

last things

My sister and I step briskly out of the greengrocer to get away from the men behind us in line who have told us, in great detail, what they'd like to do to us, where they intend to put certain parts of their bodies. The clerk, kindly, rings their purchases up slowly, so Cyndy and I have a chance to hurry across the street, almost bumping into two men who are breaking raw eggs in their hands and leaning over to slip the viscous mess into their mouths.

One of those Manhattan nights, I think.

Earlier today, as Cyndy and I were taxiing away from Grand Central to her apartment in Chelsea, we were thrilled, saying: "New York. It's so great. Look at the dirt! Look at the guy peeing in the alley! I love it!" A joke, sure, but only partially. We'd just spent a claustrophobic weekend with our parents and other two siblings in the Berkshires. The occasion, I guess, was Cyndy's mastectomy last week.

Cyndy's nerves are pretty much gone in the right side of her body, so the operation didn't hurt as much as the lumpectomy she had two years ago, when she was twenty-one. Still, I can't help thinking, Wound, especially now that we're out with the crazies. And also, I'm thinking of my own toes, which are so black and blue with cold (a circulatory problem, I will learn later in the month) that I am having trouble walking. Indeed, at the moment, I feel more damaged than Cyndy appears to feel. We shuffle by the guys with the eggs, and I put my right arm around Cyndy's back—companionably, I think, because I want to restore the playful order that has reigned most of today, that was operative when we were at New York City Opera, and I was meeting Cyndy's co-workers and admiring the Mr. Potato Head doll she had placed over her desk, presumably to supervise her efforts as rehearsals coordinator. My arm has barely touched Cyndy's black coat (the coat I will someday wear) when she says, vicious as possible, "Don't you *dare* try to protect me."

I am quiet—my throat, for a minute, as pained as my toes—and then I say, my voice strangulated, half the words swallowed, ". . . not trying . . . protect you."

Cyndy is dead, of course. That is why I wear her black coat now. She died of breast cancer at age twenty-six, a fact that I find unbelievable, a fact that is (virtually) statistically impossible. When she was twenty-one, she was in the shower in her dorm room at the University of Pennsylvania. She was washing under her arm when she found the lump. She was not checking for breast cancer. What college girl does monthly exams on her own breasts? Laura, my twin sister, says that I was the first person Cyndy called about the cancer. I don't think this is true, though Laura insists. I'm certain Cyndy called my father, the doctor, and that he told her to fly home to Boston. He demanded her return even though the doctors at Penn's health service pooh-poohed her concern. Finally, after a long conversation, I realize why Laura thinks Cyndy called me first, and I tell her: "I think you're thinking about the rape."

"Oh, yeah," Laura says. "That's probably right."

When my father called me in Wisconsin to tell me about Cyndy, I said, "Oh, well, I'm sure, she's okay. Lots of women have fibrous breasts."

"No, Debra," my father said, sternly. "That's not what this is about."

"Do you think she'll have to have a biopsy?"

He was quiet.

"A mastectomy?"

"That's the least of my concerns."

I guess I wasn't quite able to hear him right then. I hung up the phone and pulled out my copy of *Our Bodies, Ourselves* to look at that book's photograph of a jubilant naked woman—out in the sun, with one breast gone, the stitches running up her chest like a sideways zipper. I remember wailing, literally wailing, at the image and at the prospect of my sister losing her breast.

I didn't know yet that my father had examined my sister when she came home from college. My father is an endocrinologist, a fertility specialist. He examines women every day in his office, but to feel your adult daughter's breast—breaking *that* taboo, because medical care is shoddy and you *do* love your daughter desperately and *appropriately*—and to know, right away, what it is you are feeling . . . I have to stop myself from imagining it. And I think my father has to disremember it, too, because even though he knew, right then, she had cancer, he tells this story about himself: When the X ray of Cyndy's chest was up on the lightboard, my father pulled the X ray off the board and turned it over to look at the name. "Spark, C." He looked back at the picture. Turned the X ray over again to check the name. "Spark, C." He did the whole thing again. And again.

Later, two weeks before she did die, I remember seeing her X ray up on a lightboard. Not something I was supposed to see, I know, but Cyndy's treatment all took place at the same hospital my father has worked at for twenty-five years. I knew my way about and I knew how to take silent advantage when I needed to. I looked, but from a distance. I was out in the hall, standing over Cyndy in her gurney, as orderlies were about to move her out of the emergency ward and up to a floor. My view was oblique, and once I knew there was nothing happy to see there, I said, Don't look. Though later, all I would do was say, Look, Debra. Look, this is a person dying. Look, this is Cyndy going away.

My mother was always the most pessimistic of all of us, and I used to hate her for it. "She'll be okay," I'd say. And, "We can't read the future." My mother said we were lucky we *couldn't* read the future or we'd never get through it. Which is probably true. That night in Manhattan, things seemed tragic but manageable. In the past was the lumpectomy and the radiation. Now, the mastectomy was completed. The chemo was to come. Cyndy had cut her hair short so the loss of it wouldn't be too upsetting. Back in Boston, she'd gone with my mother to buy a wig. Now, she was trying to wear it over her hair. That was the advice she had been given: to start wearing it so it would be like a new haircut and no one would notice. I thought, Who cares who notices? I was for announcing the illness as just another fact, among many, about Cyndy. To keep it secret was to imply that it was either shameful, like a sin, or special, like a surprise gift, and it was neither.

The wig bothered Cyndy. It was itchy and, though we'd tell her otherwise, it had a dowdy look, a look that owed nothing to the haircuts Cyndy had always had—the funky asymmetrical do she'd sported when she'd gone to London for a year or the long red mane she'd had as a child. One day, while I was still visiting with her in New York, we went out to lunch with some friends of mine who had never met Cyndy. In the middle of lunch, Cyndy, impatient and in the midst of a story (she was a magnificent and voluble talker), pulled off her hair—to my friends' surprise, especially since there was another head of hair under the one she'd pulled off.

After all the preparation for baldness, however, Cyndy's hair didn't fall out. At least, not that year. The first round of chemo was bad, but, again, in the realm of the get-overable. Every three or four weekends, my mother would come in to New York and take Cyndy to the hospital and then out to my grandmother's house for a weekend of puking. Cyndy handled it well. The biggest long-term effect was that she wouldn't let anyone say the words "pot roast" when they were around her. And she couldn't stand the smell of toast for years to come.

Sometime later, after Cyndy had finished up the chemo, she decided to go to business school, to get a degree in arts administration at UCLA. She loved school. She had never been too happy as an undergraduate, but UCLA was right for her. Her goal had been to make opera, which she adored, accessible to people who ordinarily wouldn't go. She had a special column in the school newspaper called "Kulture, Kulture, Kulture"; she was proud of her ability to drag business students (a surprise! stiff business students!) to the opera. I imagine Cyndy as the life of the party in those days. Cyndy going to the graduate-student beer bashes, Cyndy leading the talk at the business-school study sessions, Cyndy still earning her nickname, Symphony.

I know she slimmed down in those years, too. She had an intermittent problem with her weight, and it was probably the real clue that Cyndy—handle-everything-Cyndy—sometimes had her unhealthy way of handling things. When I visited Cyndy in Chelsea, after her mastectomy, we were toying with the idea of living together. At the time, I was profoundly (read "clinically") depressed. I had left the man I had been living with for four years and had been unenthusiastically debating what I should do next. Cyndy was moving up to Inwood, and we had found a small apartment that would accommodate the two of us should I decide to move in with her. I remember that one of her real enthusiasms about the two of us living together had to do with food. She was convinced that I'd have her eating large green salads for dinner, that my own good habits would rub off on her, and she would no longer find herself in the middle of secret, ruinously upsetting food binges.

Cyndy had been a chubby kid, but never really fat, even when she weighed a lot. When she was older, her figure was sensual if robust. Still, her weight was an occasional issue: my father telling her, at dinner, not to be a *chazar,* my mother spinning her own anxiety about weight onto Cyndy. At Cyndy's graduation, Cyndy said "No, thank you" to the dessert tray that a waiter was offering our table. We were all too full. My mother said, "Oh, I'm so proud of you," to Cyndy. Cyndy said to the waiter, "I'll have that chocolate cake." And the rest of the children—Laura, David, and I—hooted with laughter. It was our turn to be proud. After all, the request for cake was her version of "Oh, stop it, Mom."

Still, toward the end of Cyndy's stay in Chelsea, I got my first glimpse of how painful the problem with food could be. Like many women, I had my own issues, and Cyndy and I would often have long talks about what all this meant. Once, she told me about how she used to have a secret way of slipping cookies silently out of the cookie jar and hiding under the dining room table to eat. This might have struck me as funny—so often our childhood stories charmed me—but I wanted to sob when she told me. I felt stricken, but stricken by our—her, my, everybody's—desires. How easily they became desperate or grotesque or hateful, especially to the person who did all that desiring.

Her desires must have been met in L.A., however, because she looked so good. At the end of her first year there, she organized a student show, a big, campy celebration that everyone dressed for. She brought a videotape of the show back to Boston for the rest of us to see. Now, we fast-forward through the tape so we can see the intermission. Someone has filmed her—happy her—backstage exuberantly organizing things. Then we fast-forward again and there is Cyndy in a gorgeous, retro, off-the-shoulder dress. Her hair is long, just above her shoulders. She needs to flip it out of her eyes. She has long dangling earrings. She is glamorous by anyone's account and quite sexy. By this point, she's had reconstructive surgery. The new breast is lumpy and disappointing—not that anyone says this. It's just clear that when my uncle, the surgeon, said, "Sometimes they do such a good job you can't tell the difference," he wasn't 100 percent correct. Part of the problem is that Cyndy, like all the women in the family, has large breasts. They couldn't reconstruct her breast so it would be as big as the original one, so she had a smaller breast made, and she wore a partial prosthesis. The doctors had asked her if she wanted the other breast reduced—for balance's sake. But she decided no. After all, she didn't want to run the risk of not having feeling in either breast.

In the videotape, when Cyndy starts to sing, the audience is clearly amazed. And they should be: her voice is stunning. She could have had an operatic career if she had wanted it. Months before her death, a singing instructor made it clear to Cyndy that she not only could, but she had to, have a singing career. Her voice was that beautiful.

Now, when I listen to the tape, I watch Cyndy's mannerisms. Each time, I am surprised by the fact that she seems a little nervous about performing. Cyndy nervous? Cyndy is never nervous, as she herself will admit. (Except about men. That's the one exception.) But she gets comfortable as she proceeds, as the audience's approval is clear. She sings, beautifully, the Carole King song "Way over Yonder." *Way over yonder, that's where I'm bound.*

Even before she died, I knew the irony would always break my heart, once she was gone.

In the summer after Cyndy's first two semesters in L.A., I was living in Lincoln, Nebraska. I was teaching a summer class, and late at night, I'd get tearful calls from Cyndy. Mostly about men, for I was, in many things, Cyndy's confidante. Sometimes, now, I think that I am wrong about this. I *was* Cyndy's confidante, wasn't I? She *was* the person who I was closest to, wasn't she?

When we were young, I always thought that Cyndy and I belonged together, and David and Laura belonged together. Laura always had a special way with David. Laura and I were close (the twins, after all), and Cyndy and David (the youngest) were playmates. Still, I felt Cyndy and I were a pair. When they met Cyndy, people used to say, "Oh, so she's your twin?" And I'd shake my head no. "Your older sister?" No, I'd say again. Cyndy loved being mistaken for my older sister. "I really am the smartest one in the family," she'd say, even when she was in her twenties. I'd have to disagree; it was a distinction I thought I deserved if by smart you meant (and Cyndy did) commonsensical.

Our closeness was somewhat competitive. We delighted in being competent—more competent than the one in the family who was spacey, the one who was overemotional. We just had things together, and we understood the world. The one fight I remember us having (I'm sure we had many when we were young, but I can't remember them) is about driving the car. She snapped at me for correcting her driving. She hated it when I played older sister.

When Cyndy first started making her tearful phone calls to me, I was proud. I took a secret pleasure in the fact that she confided in me, that she came to me first. I'd even felt a slight pleasure—mixed with horror—when she called to tell me, and, at first, only me, that she'd been raped. It was during her first year at college. I was in my senior year at Yale. It was a date rape, I suppose, although that term doesn't fit exactly. The man was someone she met in a bar—a sailor, good God—and Cyndy got drunk, and later, after some flirting, he didn't understand that no meant no. I honestly don't think he knew he raped her. I think for a while Cyndy was bewildered, too. Her previous sexual encounters had not amounted to much, and, later in college, her experiences remained disappointing.

Given her history, Cyndy's tears on the phone made sense to me. I thought she was finally addressing the issue that had always so frightened her. She spoke, with uncharacteristic frustration, of the way her women friends were always talking about *their* relationships, and that she didn't have any relationships and how upset it made her. With the encouragement of the family, Cyndy started talking to a therapist. I was all for this, I would tell Cyndy, as I sat late at night in my small rental in Nebraska. After all, I had been helped, enormously, by a psychiatrist. My parents agreed with my assessment, I think, although Cyndy spent less of her time on the phone with them talking about men and more time talking about her headaches, her terrible headaches that stopped her from getting any work done.

So, it's clear where this goes, no? We hope it's not, we hope it's not—as with each test or checkup, we have hoped—but it is. Cyndy has cancer in her brain. When they do the initial radiation on her brain, and later when they do an experimental treatment that *does* shrink the tumor, it becomes clear that all that crying had a physiological base. Her tumor shrunk, her headaches go away. She stops crying or talking about men.

But, of course, she does cry, though only once, when she learns about the brain tumor. When I find out, I am standing in my kitchen and kneading bread. I get the call, and then I phone MIT to tell a friend of Laura's not to let her go to lunch. I want to come get her and take her to the hospital. I feel like a rock when I do all this, like a cold rock. I throw the dough into the trash and hear the *thump-swish* of it hitting the plastic bag. Then, I go and get Laura, who screams—as in bad movies, screams—and I drive to the hospital. Laura, instantly feeling everything, spins out of control with grief. She's sharp with nurses who seem to be blocking her way to Cyndy. She won't allow what my father says when he says it. She just tells him, No, no, you're wrong. She turns to me and says, Why aren't you acting like anything? And I think, Because I am so very competent.

. . .

In the fall, Cyndy comes and lives with me in my big apartment in North Cambridge. This is so clearly better than staying with my parents in their suburban home. She is immensely disappointed about having to take time off from UCLA. But it is only time off, we reassure her. She will get back there. And she does. After a year with me, she goes back for a semester. But she is too sick and has to come back to live with me for good. She lives with me for two years. This is the part that I'm glad I didn't get to see when I was in my Wisconsin apartment and worrying about the possibility of my sister having a mastectomy. I think now, A mastectomy! A lousy mastectomy! Who cares? I remember once, not long after I'd moved to Cambridge and before Cyndy moved in with me, I was in bed with a temporary lover. He was an old college friend, a doctor, in town to do some work for the year. Cyndy and I had been talking, earlier that day, over the phone, about men. I was encouraging her to approach a young man she was interested in, in L.A. She'd said, "But, it's so complicated. Like at what point do I say, 'Hey, buddy. One of these isn't real.'" I knew she'd be gesturing, even though we were on the phone, to her chest, pointing to first one, then the other. ("I can always tell," she'd said, "when someone knows and they're trying to figure out which one it is.") That night, in bed, I'd said to my friend, "Well, if you loved someone, it wouldn't make a difference . . . say, before you were involved . . . if you found out they had a mastectomy, would it?" He looked at me. "Yeah," he said. "I don't mean to be horrible, but of course it would."

"But," I said, as if he'd change his mind because I needed him to, "*I* said it wouldn't. That's what *I* said."

Cyndy and I had fun in the apartment where we lived. My boyfriend, Jim, would come by in the evenings, and they would talk music or we'd go out for dinner. Nights when Jim was working, we'd get George, a musician friend from around the corner, to come over. Cyndy took classes at Boston University. She worked for the Boston Opera Theatre. She got involved with a project involving musicians in Prague. Related to that, Václav Havel's press secretary and her son came to live with us for a while. And during all this, cancer would pop up in one place or another—her knees, the back of her tongue. Still, it always honestly seemed to me that we could make her better. Healthy denial, I suppose. Certainly, Cyndy had a lot of it. She was always willing to be cheered up, to imagine her future.

Some things stand out, but I can't (I won't) put them in order. Like: the number of times I would be in bed, making love with Jim, and hear Cyndy hacking away in the next room. That would be the cancer in her lungs.

Or the way she would call out to me each morning that Jim wasn't there: "Derba, Derba, Derba," she'd say, in a high-pitched silly voice. And I'd call back, "Der-ba Bird," because that was what she was, chirping out the family nickname for me. Then, I'd go crawl into her bed and rub her back. There was cancer in the spine by then, and she could never get comfortable. Sometimes, she'd wail at her pillows. She couldn't get them in the right position.

Or the way, one night, when I was making dinner, she said, "Oh, God," and I said, "What is it?" and she snapped, angry as could be, "You *know* what it is!"

There was an odd stretch when I felt her oncologist was trying to convince her that her symptoms were psychosomatic. Like when she couldn't get enough energy to move, and we'd spend days inside, only making an occasional trek to the back porch. Perhaps, he seemed to be suggesting, she was only depressed?

The few times Cyndy did snap at me, I felt like I would dissolve. My mother said, "Well, I guess you're getting a sense, before your time, of what it's like to have an adolescent." In truth, my mother got the brunt of it. When Cyndy was in the most pain, she would leave the apartment for a stay with my parents. When she was well enough, she would come back to stay with me. Wherever she was, though—my house, my parents' house—we were all there, all the time.

And even when she was doing relatively well, there were lots of visits back and forth. One day, in the beginning of her stay with me, Cyndy and I were driving out to our parents' house for dinner. We were talking about death, and Cyndy said, "Oh, well, you know, sometimes I think about death. And I try to force myself to imagine what it would be like but then I'm like . . . whoa . . . you know, I just can't do it."

"Yes," I said, for I knew exactly what she meant. "I'm like that, too."

Now I'm even more "like that." For if a parent's job is to protect his or her child, a sister's is to identify with her sibling. Which means, of course, that the whole family gets, in the case of a terminal illness, to fail in what they most want to do for one another. So I push my imagination to death, make myself think, No consciousness. I have, regretfully, no belief in heaven, an afterlife, reincarnation. I believe in nothingness. I try not to let myself pull back, try not to say, "Whoa, that's too much." But my brain—its gift to me—is that it won't let me do what I want.

I think, in this regard, of the time ten-year-old Cyndy came home from school in a snit. She'd learned about black holes in science class. She'd stomped up to her room and flopped onto her bed. As she climbed the stairs, she ordered the family never to talk to her about black holes. I thought she was joking. So, I opened the door to her bedroom, stuck my head in—cartoon fashion, the accordion player poking his head through the stage curtain to get a peek at the crowd—and I said, rapidly, "Black hole, black hole, black hole." Cyndy, already lying on her bed, threw herself against the mattress so that she bounced on it like a just-captured fish hitting land. She started to sob. "I'm sorry," I said. "I was kidding. I thought *you* were kidding." But why should she have been? What's more terrible than everything going out?

Once, during one of her final stays in the hospital, Cyndy said to my mother, "I'm going to be good now," as if that would make her healthy, as if a planet could blame itself for being in the wrong part of the universe.

"Oh, honey," my mother had said, "You *are* good. You are so *good*."

One trip out to my parents that stands in my mind: Cyndy had the shingles, an enormously painful viral infection that runs along the nerve path on one side of the body. Just getting her down the staircase into my car was horrible. Cyndy was sobbing and sobbing, and ordinarily she didn't cry. I put her in the passenger's seat and cursed myself for having the kind of life that made me buy such an inexpensive and uncomfortable car. The requirement of bending was too much, and Cyndy wept and wept. I drove as fast as I could and neither of us talked. I thought, I'll just get her home and it will be all right. My father, the doctor, would know what to do. My mother would be, as she could be, the most comforting person in the world. When we got there, I said, "It's okay, it's going to be okay," as Cyndy walked, with tiny paces, from the car to the front steps. My parents were at the front door and it was night. My mother brought a kitchen chair to the front hall so as soon as Cyndy got up the stairs, she could sit down. I stood behind her, and my parents stood at the top of the six stairs that lead to our front door. My mother (blue turtleneck and jeans), my father (stooped). Both of them had their hands out and were reaching for Cyndy but they couldn't get her up the stairs. She had to do that herself. And I thought, looking at them in the light, and Cyndy still forcing herself up through the night—*Oh, my God. All this love, all this love can't do a thing.*

But that wasn't completely true. The love did do something. It just didn't save her.

Laura, my twin sister, gave Cyndy foot rubs and Cyndy loved them. Laura would give foot rubs, literally, for hours. I gave back rubs but I never liked giving them, would wait for Cyndy to say I could stop. When Cyndy told Laura she could stop if she wanted to,

Laura would ask for permission to keep going—as if Cyndy were doing her a favor by putting her feet in the vicinity of Laura's hands. One day, Cyndy was lying on her bed in our apartment and Laura was on a chair at the end of the bed and she was rubbing Cyndy's feet. I was "spooning" Cyndy and occasionally rubbing up and down her spine where the cancer was. We were talking about masturbation. "I can't believe you guys," Laura was saying, telling us again about how amazing it was that of the three of us, she had discovered masturbation first. We were giggling. This conversation wasn't unfamiliar. We'd had it before, but we could always find something new to tell each other.

"What was that bathtub thing you were talking about," Cyndy said.

Years earlier, I'd instructed both of my sisters about the virtues of masturbating in the bathtub. Something I'd learned from my freshman-year roommate at college. "Got to try it," I said now.

"Exactly how do you do it again?" asked Cyndy.

"Lie in the tub. Scoot your butt under the waterspout and put your legs up on the wall and let the water run into you. Guaranteed orgasm."

"De-bra," Cyndy said, hitting me, as if I'd gone too far in this being-open-with-sisters conversation.

"Sor-ry," I said. "Still, you've got to try it, but wait till this thing gets better." I pointed to her head. There was a new problem these days, something that caused Cyndy to get, on occasions, dizzy. She had some new medicine, so I talked as if the problem would be solved in a matter of weeks. (Aside from the dizziness, Cyndy had occasional aphasia. One night when I was on the phone, Cyndy screamed from her bedroom. I ran in. She'd forgotten a word, couldn't produce it, and felt her head go weirdly blank. The word, she realized, five minutes later, was cancer.)

We decided to leave the topic of sex behind for something else. But not before I insisted, once again, that Cyndy try this bathtub thing. I was rubbing her back and Laura was still rubbing her feet, and I was thinking, as I stroked her skin, Yes, an orgasm. Let this body give her some pleasure.

You *do* get inappropriately intimate with a body when the body is ill. Sometimes there's something nice about it. Cyndy used to sit on the toilet in our bathroom and I'd take a soapy washcloth and wash her bald head. I'd say, "Stamp out dry scalpy skin." This struck us, for some reason, as terribly funny. We'd soak our feet in the bathtub and talk about our favorite Gogol stories. We'd walk arm in arm. Say: "This is what we'll be like when we are old ladies."

When Cyndy's symptoms were at their worst, my own body struck me, especially my legs, which stretched—it seemed amazing—from my torso to the ground. The miracle of walking. I still feel it. The air behind my legs is creepily light as I move. Who would have ever suspected that you can feel grief behind your kneecaps?

One very bad night: Cyndy was upset about everything, but especially men, relationships, never having had a boyfriend. According to her, I didn't, *couldn't* understand because I had had a boyfriend. This was a point of connection between Cyndy and a few of her intimates, an absence they could discuss and from which I was excluded. It didn't matter that I felt, for the sadness of my own relationships, included. I had had sex. Many times even—enough to have had a sexually transmitted disease, which I (paranoid, irrational) thought I could pass on to Cyndy through ordinary contact. It didn't matter that I was cured of the problem. Her immune system was down. Anything I did might hurt her. My own desires might kill her.

This one night, Cyndy was crying, so I went into her room to

put my arm around her, and she said, "Don't. Don't you touch me."
Fierce again. Vicious. I retreated to my bedroom. Cried softly, but
still felt I had to do something. I stepped back to her bedroom, and
she started to scream, waving me away, but saying, "It's just that I
realize that nobody but my family or a doctor has touched me in the
past five years."

It'll change, it'll change, it'll change. That was always my
mantra for these relationship conversations. But it didn't. She died
before it could change.

After that terrible night when Cyndy had the shingles and had to
struggle out of our apartment to the car, she spent six weeks at my
parents' house. Those were miserable times. She couldn't move
from her bed. We'd all climb onto the double bed, a ship in the
ocean of her room, and play word games or watch TV or be quiet
because a lot of the time she couldn't stand for anything to be going
on. As she started to feel a bit better, she worked on the course that
she was going to teach in January of 1992. It was going to be called
Opera—What's All the Screaming About? and it was going to be
for high school girls, for kids who, presumably, couldn't care less
about opera. We rented opera videos and watched them with her.
Then, she decided she was ready to come back to our apartment to
work on her course syllabus. I cleaned the kitchen while she worked.
At one point, she started to faint, but she grabbed the doorjamb, and
I came in and caught her, wrapped my arms around her waist—big
now, she was bloated with steroids—and set her down on the
ground. She was okay, so she started to work at her computer, and I
made us some cocoa. She handed me her syllabus to proofread. She
sipped, while I read it, and she said, in a sort of campy voice,
"Mmmm . . . this is love-ly." I laughed, still reading. She made a
funny gurgling noise. I thought it was joke but when I looked up
from the syllabus, Cyndy was slipping out of her chair. I ran the few

feet to her. She was crumpled on the ground. I rolled her onto her back and saw blood. There was water on the floor—her urine. "Are you okay? Are you okay?" I screamed. Her wig had rolled off her head and she looked like a gigantic toppled mannequin. She was gasping, breathing oddly. A seizure, I knew. I am, after all, a doctor's daughter. When the convulsive breathing stopped, she said, "What happened? What just happened?" She was as purely frightened as I'd ever seen her.

"Close your eyes," I said. "You just fainted. Close your eyes." I didn't want her to see her own blood. I thought that would scare her. I ran to the bathroom to get a towel and wipe her up. I tried to see where the blood was coming from.

"It's okay, you bit your tongue."

I felt—I have to say this, only because it's so horrible—a slight pleasure. It was the old thing; I would be competent, take care of this trouble. I was good in an emergency. But, there was also part of me—small, I promise myself now, very small—that thought, with some relief, It's over.

The ambulance came. We rode over to the hospital. My parents were there before us. When they rolled Cyndy away, I cried to my mother, "Oh, Mommy. I thought she was dying. I thought she was dying."

Inside, Cyndy was saying the same to my father, "I thought I was dying. I thought I was going to die."

And about two weeks later she did. But not before her body put her through enormous suffering. Not before she had a little more fun with the family. So, last things. The last thing she ever produced was a picture from a coloring book. She had asked for the book and some crayons, and we all earnestly filled in Mickey Mouse's ears and then signed our names and ages. Debra, twenty-nine. Laura, twenty-nine. David, twenty-four. Mommy, fifty-three. Daddy, fifty-five. Cyndy signed hers, "The Queen." (A joke from our two years together. When she was queen, Boston drivers were not going to be allowed to be obnoxious.) Under "age," Cyndy wrote, "None of your damn business." Last meal: gray fish from the kosher kitchen, but she didn't eat it. Last thing she *did* eat: Jell-O. I know, I spooned it into her mouth. Last thing I said to her: I told her that the man she was interested in was in love with her, that I knew because of what he'd said when I called to tell him she was in the hospital. (I was making this up, but who cares?) Last thing Cyndy ever said to me: "Oh, good. Well, tell him we'll get together when I get out of here." Last thing she ever said: I didn't hear this because I wasn't in the room, but she woke up, delusional and panicked and worried because she was going on a long trip and she hadn't packed her suitcase.

As my fiction-writer friends always say, You can't make this stuff up. No one would believe you if you tried.

And I have to agree: real life is just too heavy handed.

Very last thing: her body still desiring life, she takes every third breath, though her fingers are dusky, though her kidneys have already shut down. We give the funeral director the pretty purple dress she bought for special occasions. We put her in the ground.

Our desires, I sometimes think now, as I'm walking down the street. Today, outside a bakery, I stop myself and say, Yes, Debra? What about them? And I realize I don't know. What? What? I stand for a while feeling disgusted with the world—those horrible leering men in the greengrocer's; that stupid sailor in the bar; foolish me, making love with my sister dying in the next room. *Our desires, our desires, our desires.* I know what the refrain is; I just don't know what to do about it. It's a reproach for me, an always unfulfilled wish for my family, and a sad song—it's a dirge—for Cyndy. Still, since I am here, stuck among the living, I have to remind myself that the song owes nothing to the beautiful ones that Cyndy sang. So I go into the bakery and get a shortbread cookie, dipped in chocolate. It is so delicious I start to cry.

oliver sacks

Oliver Sacks's profile of Dr. Bennett, a surgeon with Tourette's syndrome, is simultaneously factual and informative—and very cinematic. There are eight strong scenes offering dialogue, description, and revealing detail. Sacks is authoritative and personal, effectively responding to and interacting with Bennett without self-indulgence. The defining moment is when Sacks, the writer/observer, must become a vital part of the narrative and demonstrate faith in his subject by entrusting Bennett with his own life.

a neurologist's notebook:
a surgeon's life

Tourette's syndrome is seen in every race, every culture, every stratum of society; it can be recognized at a glance once one is attuned to it; and cases of barking and twitching, of grimacing, of strange gesturing, of involuntary cursing and blaspheming were recorded by Aretaeus of Cappadocia almost two thousand years ago. Yet it was not clinically delineated until 1885, when Georges Gille de la Tourette, a young French neurologist—a pupil of Charcot's, and a friend of Freud's—put together these historical accounts with observations of some of his own patients. The syndrome as he described it was characterized, above all, by convulsive tics, by involuntary mimicry or repetition of others' words or actions (echolalia and echopraxia), and by the involuntary or compulsive utterances of curses and obscenities (coprolalia). Some individuals (despite their affliction) showed an odd insouciance or nonchalance; some a tendency to make strange, often witty, occasionally dreamlike associations; some extreme impulsiveness and provocativeness, a constant testing of physical and social boundaries; some a constant, restless reacting to the environment, a lunging at and sniffing of everything, or a sudden flinging of objects; and yet others an extreme stereotypy and obsessiveness—no two patients were ever quite the same.

Any disease introduces a doubleness into life—an "it," with its own needs, demands, limitations. With Tourette's, the "it" takes the form of explicit compulsion, of a multitude of explicit compulsions: one is driven to do this, to do that, against one's will. Tourette's may seize control at any time. Being "taken over" or "possessed" can be more than a figure of speech for someone with severe Tourette's, and no doubt in the Middle Ages Tourette's was sometimes seen as "possession." (Tourette himself was fascinated by the phenomenon of "possession" and wrote a play about the epidemic of demonic possession in medieval Loudun.)

But the relation of disease and self, "it" and "I," can be particularly complex in Tourette's, especially if it has been present from early childhood, growing up with the self, intertwining itself in every possible way. The Tourette's and the self shape themselves each to the other, come more and more to complement each other, until finally, like a long-married couple, they become a single, compound being. This relation is often destructive, but it can also be constructive, can add speed and spontaneity, and a capacity for unusual and sometimes startling performance. For all its intrusiveness, Tourette's may be used creatively, too.

Yet in the years after its first delineation, Tourette's tended to be seen not as an organic but as a "moral" disease—an expression of mischievousness or weakness of the will, to be treated by rectifying the will. From the 1920s to the 1960s, it tended to be seen as a psychiatric disease, to be treated by psychoanalysis or psychotherapy; but this, on the whole, proved ineffective, too. Then, with the demonstration, in the early sixties, that the drug haloperidol could dramatically suppress its symptoms, Tourette's was regarded—in a sudden reversal—as a chemical disease, the result of an imbalance of a neurotransmitter, dopamine, in the brain. But all these views are partial, and reductive, and fail to do justice to the full complexity of Tourette's, which may be almost as complex as human nature itself. Neither a biological nor a psychological nor a moral-social viewpoint is adequate; we must see Tourette's simultaneously from all three perspectives—as a biopsychosocial disorder. And one that is far from uncommon: it affects perhaps one person in a thousand.

Many professions, one would think, would be closed to someone with elaborate tics and compulsions, but this does not seem to be the case. We find people with Tourette's—sometimes the most severe Tourette's—in virtually every walk of life. There are Tourettic writers, mathematicians, musicians, actors, disc jockeys, construction workers, mechanics, athletes. Some things, one might think, would be completely out of the question—above all, perhaps, the intricate, precise, and steady work of a surgeon. This would have been my own belief not so long ago. But now, improbably, I know *five* surgeons with Tourette's.

I first met Dr. Carl Bennett, as I will call him, at a scientific conference on Tourette's in Boston last year. His appearance was unexceptionable—he was fiftyish, of middle size, with a brownish beard and mustache containing a hint of gray, and was dressed soberly in a dark suit—until he suddenly lunged or reached for the ground or jumped or jerked. I was struck both by his bizarre tics and by his dignity and calm. When I expressed incredulity about his choice of profession, he invited me to visit and stay with him, where he lived and practiced, in a town that I will call Branford, in British Columbia—to do rounds at the hospital with him, to scrub with him, to see him in action. Now, four months later, in early October, I found myself in a small plane approaching Branford, full of curiosity and mixed expectations. Dr. Bennett met me at the airport, greeted me—a strange greeting, half-lunge, half-tic; a gesture of welcome idiosyncratically Tourettized—grabbed my case, and led the way to his car in an odd, rapid skipping walk, with a skip each fifth step and sudden reachings to the ground as if to pick something up.

The situation of Branford is almost idyllic, nestled as it is in the shadow of the Rockies, in southeast British Columbia, with Banff and its mountains to the north, and Montana and Idaho to the south; it lies in a region of great gentleness and fertility but ringed with mountains, glaciers, lakes. Bennett himself has a passion for geography and geology; a few years ago he took a year off from his surgical practice to study both at the University of Victoria. As he drove, he pointed out moraines, stratifications, and other formations, so that what had at first seemed to my eyes a mere pastoral landscape became charged with a sense of history and chthonic forces, of immense geological vistas. Such keen, fierce attention to every detail, such constant looking below the surface, such examination and analysis, is characteristic of the restless, questioning Tourettic mind. It is, so to speak, the other side of its obsessive and perseverative tendencies, its disposition to reiterate, to touch again and again.

And, indeed, whenever the stream of attention and interest was interrupted, Bennett's tics and iterations immediately reasserted themselves—in particular, obsessive touchings of his mustache and glasses. His mustache had constantly to be smoothed and checked for symmetry, his glasses had to be "balanced"—up and down, side to side, diagonally, in and out—with sudden, ticcy touchings of the fingers, until these, too, were exactly "centered." There were also occasional reachings and lungings of his right arm; sudden, compulsive touchings of the windshield with both forefingers ("The touching has to be symmetrical," he commented); sudden repositionings of his knees, or the steering wheel ("I have to have the knees symmetrical in relation to the steering wheel. They have to be *exactly* centered"); and sudden, high-pitched vocalizations, in a voice completely unlike his own, that sounded like "Hi, Patty," "Hi, there," and, on a couple of occasions, "Hideous!" (Patty, I learned later, was a former girlfriend, her name now enshrined in a tic.)

There was little hint of this repertoire until we reached town and got obstructed by traffic lights. The lights did not annoy Bennett—we were in no hurry—but they did break up the driving, the kinetic melody, the swift, smooth stream of action, with its power to integrate mind and brain. The transition was very sudden: one minute, all was smoothness and action; the next, all was broken-upness, pandemonium, riot. When Bennett was driving smoothly, one had the feeling not that the Tourette's was in any way being suppressed but that the brain and the mind were in a quite different mode of action.

Another few minutes, and we had arrived at his house, a charming, idiosyncratic house with a wild garden, perched on a hill overlooking the town. Bennett's dogs, rather wolflike, with strange, pale eyes, barked, wagged their tails, bounded up to us as we drove in. As we got out of the car, he said "Hi, puppies!" in the same quick, odd, high, crushed voice he had earlier used for "Hi, Patty!" He patted their heads, a ticlike, convulsive patting, a quick-fire volley of five pats to each, delivered with a meticulous symmetry and synchrony. "They're grand dogs, half Eskimo, half malamute," he said. "I felt I should get two of them, so they could companion each other. They play together, sleep together, hunt together—everything." And, I thought, are patted together: did he get two dogs partly because of his own symmetrical, symmetrizing compulsions? Now, hearing the dogs bark, his sons ran out—two handsome teenage kids. I had a sudden feeling that Bennett might cry "Hi, kiddies!" in his Touretty voice, and pat their heads, too, in synchrony, symmetrically. But he introduced them, Mark and David, individually to me. And then, as we entered the house, he introduced me to his wife, Helen, who was preparing a late-afternoon tea for all of us.

As we sat at the table, Bennett was repeatedly distracted by tics—a compulsive touching of the glass lampshade above his head. He had to tap the glass gently with the nails of both forefingers, to produce a sharp, half musical click or, on occasion, a short salvo of clicks. A third of his time was taken up with this ticcing and clicking, which he seemed unable to stop. Did he have to do it? Did he have to sit there?

"If it were out of reach, would you still have to click it?" I asked.

"No," he said. "It depends entirely on how I'm situated. It's all a question of space. Where I am now, for example, I have no impulse to reach over to that brick wall, but if I were in range I'd have to touch it perhaps a hundred times." I followed his glance to the wall, and saw that it was pockmarked, like the moon, from his touchings and jabbings; and, beyond it, the refrigerator door, dented and battered, as if from the impact of meteorites or projectiles. "Yeah," Bennett said, now following my glance. "I fling things—the iron, the rolling pin, the saucepan, whatever—I fling things at it if I suddenly get enraged." I digested this information in silence. It added a new dimension—a disquieting, violent one—to the picture I was building and seemed completely at odds with the genial, tranquil man before me.

"If the light so disturbs you, why do you sit near it?" I asked.

"Sure, it's 'disturbance,'" Bennett answered. "But it's also stimulation. I like the feel and the sound of the 'click.' But, yeah, it can be a great distraction. I can't study here, in the dining room—I have to go to my study, out of reach of the lamp."

Another expression of his Tourette's—very different from the sudden impulsive or compulsive touching—is a slow, almost sensuous pressing of the foot to mark out a circle in the ground all around him. "It seems to me almost instinctual," he said when I asked him about it. "Like a dog marking its territory. I feel it in my bones. I think it is something primal, prehuman—maybe something that all of us, without knowing it, have in us. But Tourette's 'releases' these primitive behaviors."

Bennett sometimes calls Tourette's "a disease of disinhibition." He says there are thoughts not unusual in themselves that anyone might have in passing but are normally inhibited. With him, such thoughts perseverate in the back of the mind, obsessively, and burst out suddenly, without his consent or intention. Thus, he says, when the weather is nice he may want to be out in the sun getting a tan. This thought will be in the back of his mind while he is seeing his patients in the hospital and will emerge in sudden, involuntary utterances. "The nurse may say, 'Mr. Jones has abdominal pain,' and I'm looking out of the window saying, 'Tanning rays, tanning rays.' It might come out five hundred times in a morning. People in the ward must hear it—they can't *not* hear it—but I guess they ignore it, or feel that it doesn't matter."

Sometimes the Tourette's manifests itself in obsessive thoughts and anxieties. "If I'm worried about something," Bennett told me as we sat around the table, "say, I hear a story about a kid being hurt, I have to go up and tap the wall and say, 'I hope it won't happen to mine.'" I witnessed this for myself a couple of days later. There was a news report on TV about a lost child, which distressed and agitated him. He instantly began touching his glasses (top, bottom, left, right, top, bottom, left, right), centering and recentering them in a fury. He made "whoo, whoo" noises, like an owl, and muttered sotto voce, "David, David—is *he* all right?" Then he dashed from the room to make sure. There was an intense anxiety and overconcern; an immediate alarm at the mention of any lost or hurt child; an immediate identification with himself, with his own children; an immediate, superstitious need to check up.

After tea, Bennett and I went out for a walk, past a little orchard heavy with apples, and on up the hill overlooking the town, the friendly malamutes gamboling around us. As we walked, he told me something of his life. He did not know whether anyone in his family had Tourette's—he was an adopted child. His own Tourette's had started when he was seven. "As a kid, growing up in Toronto, I wore glasses, I had bands on my teeth, *and* I twitched," he said. "That was the coup de grace. I kept my distance. I was a loner; I'd go for long hikes by myself. I never had friends phoning all the time, like Mark—the contrast is very great." But being a loner and taking long hikes by himself toughened him as well, made him resourceful, gave him a sense of independence and self-sufficiency. He was always good with his hands and loved the structure of natural things—the way rocks formed, the way plants grew, the way animals moved, the way muscles balanced and pulled against each other, the way the body was put together. He decided very early that he wanted to be a surgeon.

Anatomy came "naturally" to him, he said, but he found medical school extremely difficult, not merely because of his tics and touchings, which became more elaborate with the years, but because of strange difficulties and obsessions that obstructed the act of reading. "I'd have to read each line many times," he said. "I'd have to line up each paragraph to get all four corners symmetrically in my visual field." Besides this lining up of each paragraph, and sometimes of each line, he was beset by the need to "balance" syllables and words, by the need to "symmetrize" the punctuation in his mind, by the need to check the frequency of a given letter, and by the need to repeat words or phrases or lines to himself. All this made it impossible to read easily and fluently. Those problems are still with him and make it difficult for him to skim quickly, to get the gist, or to enjoy fine writing or narrative or poetry. But they did force him to read painstakingly and to learn his medical texts very nearly by heart.

When he got out of medical school, he indulged his interest in faraway places, particularly in the north: he worked as a general practitioner in the Northwest Territories and the Yukon, and he worked on icebreakers circling the Arctic. He had a gift for intimacy and grew close to the Eskimos he worked with; and he became something of an expert in polar medicine. And when he married, in 1968—he was twenty-eight—he went with his bride around the world and gratified a boyhood wish to climb Kilimanjaro.

For the past seventeen years, he has practiced in small, isolated communities in western Canada—first, for twelve years, as a general practitioner in a small city. Then, five years ago, when the need to have mountains, wild country, and lakes on his doorstep grew stronger, he moved to Branford. ("And here I will stay. I never want to leave it.") Branford, he told me, has the right "feel." The people are warm but not chummy; they keep a certain distance. There is a natural well-bredness and civility. The schools are of high quality; there is a community college, there are theaters and bookstores—Helen runs one of them—but there is also a strong feeling for the outdoors, for the wilds. There is much hunting and fishing, but Bennett prefers backpacking and climbing and cross-country skiing.

When Bennett first came to Branford, he was regarded, he thought, with a certain suspicion. "A surgeon who twitches! Who needs him? What next?" There were no patients at first, and he did not know if he could make it there, but gradually he won the town's affection and respect. His practice began to expand, and his colleagues, who had at first been startled and incredulous, soon came to trust and accept him, too, and to bring him fully into the medical community. "But enough said," he concluded as we returned to the house. It was almost dark now, and the lights of Branford were twinkling. "Come to the hospital tomorrow—we have a conference at seven-thirty. Then I'll do outpatients, and rounds on my patients. And Friday I operate—you can scrub with me."

I slept soundly in the Bennetts' basement room that night, but in the morning I woke early, roused by a strange whirring noise in the room next to mine—the playroom. The playroom door had translucent glass panels. As I peered through them, still half asleep, I saw what appeared to be a locomotive in motion—a large, whirring wheel going round and round, and giving off puffs of smoke and occasional hoots. Bewildered, I opened the door and peeked in. Bennett, stripped to the waist, was pedaling furiously on an exercise bike while calmly smoking a large pipe. A pathology book was open before him—turned, I observed, to the chapter on neurofibromatosis. This is how he invariably begins each morning—a half hour on his bike, puffing his favorite pipe, with a pathology or surgery book open to the day's work before him. The pipe, the rhythmic exercise calm him. There are no tics, no compulsions—at most, a little hooting. (He seems to imagine at such times that he is a prairie train.) He can read without his usual obsessions and distractions.

But as soon as the rhythmic cycling stopped, a flurry of tics and compulsions took over; he kept digging at his belly, which was trim, and muttering, "Fat, fat, fat . . . fat, fat, fat . . . fat, fat, fat," and then, puzzlingly, "Fat and a quarter tit." (Sometimes the "tit" was left out.)

"What does it mean?" I asked.

"I have no idea. Nor do I know where 'Hideous' comes from— it suddenly appeared one day two years ago. It'll disappear one day, and there will be another word instead. When I'm tired, it turns into

86

'Gideous.' One cannot always find sense in these words; often it is just the sound that attracts me. Any odd sound, any odd name, may start repeating itself, get me going. I get hung up with a word for two or three months. Then, one morning, it's gone, and there's another one in its place." Knowing his appetite for strange words and sounds, Bennett's sons are constantly on the lookout for "odd" names—names that sound odd to an English-speaking ear, many of them foreign. They scan the papers and their books for such words, they listen to the radio and TV, and when they find a "juicy" name, they add it to a list they keep. Bennett says of this list, "It's about the most valuable thing in the house." He calls these words "candy for the mind."

This list was started six years ago, after the name Oginga Odinga, with its alliterations, got Bennett going—and now it contains over two hundred names. Of these, twenty-two are "current" at the present time—apt to be regurgitated at any moment and chewed over, repeated, and savored internally. Of the twenty-two, the name of Slavek J. Hurka—an industrial-relations professor at the University of Saskatchewan, where Helen studies—goes the furthest back; it started to echolale itself in 1974 and has been doing so, without significant breaks, for the last seventeen years. Most words last only a few months. Some of the names (Boris Blank, Floyd Flak, Morris Good, Lubor J. Zinkl) have a short, percussive quality. Others (Yelberton A. Tittle, Babaloo Mandel) are marked by euphonious polysyllabic alliterations. It is only the sound of the words, their "melody" as Bennett says, that implants them in his mind; their origins and meanings and associations are irrelevant.

"It is similar with the number compulsions," he said. "Now I have to do everything by threes or fives, but until a few months ago it was fours and sevens. Then one morning I woke up—*four* and *seven* had gone, but *three* and *five* had appeared instead. It's as if one circuit were turned on upstairs, and another turned off. It doesn't seem to have anything to do with *me*."

At 7:25, we drove into town. It took barely five minutes to get to the hospital, but our arrival there was more complicated than usual, because Bennett had unwittingly become notorious. He had been interviewed by a magazine a few weeks earlier, and the article had just come out. Everyone was smiling and ribbing him about it. A little embarrassed, but also enjoying it, Bennett took the joking in good part. ("I'll never live it down—I'll be a marked man now.") In the doctors' common room, Bennett was clearly very much at ease with his colleagues, and they with him. One sign of this ease, paradoxically, was that he felt free to Tourette with them—to touch or tap them gently with his fingertips, or, on two occasions when he was sharing a sofa, to suddenly twist on his side and tap his colleague's shoulder with his toes—a practice I had observed in other Touretters. Bennett is somewhat cautious with his Tourettisms on first acquaintance, and conceals or downplays them until he gets to know people. When he first started working at the hospital, he told me, he would skip in the corridors only after checking to be sure that no one was looking; now when he skips or hops no one gives it a second glance.

The conversations in the common room were like those in any hospital—doctors talking among themselves about unusual cases. Bennett himself, lying half curled on the floor, kicking and thrusting one foot in the air, described an unusual case of neurofibromatosis—a young man whom he had recently operated on. His colleagues listened attentively. The abnormality of the behavior and the complete normality of the discourse formed an extraordinary contrast. There was something bizarre about the whole scene; but it was evidently so common as to be unremarkable, and no longer attracted the slightest notice. But an outsider seeing it would have been stunned.

After coffee and muffins, we repaired to the surgical outpatients department, where half a dozen patients awaited Bennett. The first was a trail guide from Banff, very western in plaid shirt, tight jeans, and cowboy hat. His horse had fallen and rolled on top of him, and he had developed an immense pseudocyst of the pancreas. Bennett spoke with the man—who said the swelling was diminishing—and gently, smoothly palpated the fluctuant mass in his abdomen. He checked the sonograms with the radiologist—they confirmed the cyst's recession—and then came back and reassured the patient. "It's going down by itself. It's shrinking nicely—you won't be needing surgery at all. You can get back to riding. I'll see you in a month." And the trail guide, delighted, walked off with a jaunty step. Later, I had a word with the radiologist. "Bennett's not only a whiz at diagnosis," he said. "He's the most compassionate surgeon I know."

The next patient was a heavy woman with a melanoma on her buttock that needed to be excised at some depth. Bennett scrubbed up, donned sterile gloves. Something about the sterile field, the prohibition, seemed to stir his Tourette's; he made sudden darting motions, or incipient motions, of his sterile, gloved right hand toward the ungloved, unwashed, "dirty" part of his left arm. The patient eyed this without expression. What did she think, I wondered, of this odd darting motion and the sudden convulsive shakings he also made with his hand? She could not have been entirely surprised, for her G.P. must have prepared her to some extent, must have said, "You need a small operation. I recommend Dr. Bennett—he's a wonderful surgeon. I have to tell you that he sometimes makes strange movements and sounds—he has a thing called Tourette's syndrome—but don't worry, it doesn't matter. It never affects his surgery."

Now, the preliminaries over, Bennett got down to the serious work, swabbing the buttock with an iodine antiseptic and then injecting local anesthetic, with an absolutely steady hand. But as soon as the rhythm of action was broken for a moment—he needed more local, and the nurse held out the vial for him to refill his syringe— there was once again the darting and near touching. The nurse did not bat an eyelid; she had seen it before and knew he wouldn't contaminate his gloves. Now, with a firm hand, Bennett made an oval incision an inch to either side of the melanoma, and in forty seconds he had removed it, along with a Brazil-nut-shaped wedge of fat and skin. "It's out!" he said. Then, very rapidly, with great dexterity, he sewed the margins of the wound together, putting five neat knots on each nylon stitch. The patient, twisting her head, watched him as he sewed, and joshed him: "Do you do all the sewing at home?"

He laughed. "Yes. All except the socks. But no one darns socks these days."

She looked again. "You're making quite a quilt."

The whole operation completed in less than three minutes, Bennett cried, "Done! Here's what we took." He held the lump of flesh before her.

"Ugh!" she exclaimed, with a shudder. "Don't show me. But thanks anyway."

All this looked highly professional from beginning to end and, apart from the dartings and near touchings, non-Tourettic. But I couldn't decide about Bennett's showing the excised lump to the patient. ("Here!") One may show a gallstone to a patient, but does one show a bleeding, misshapen piece of fat and flesh? Clearly, she didn't want to see it, but Bennett wanted to show it, and I wondered if this urge was part of his Tourettic scrupulosity and exactitude, his need to have everything looked at and understood. I had the same thought later in the morning, when he was seeing an old lady in whose bile duct he had inserted a T-tube. He went to great lengths to draw the tube, to explain all the anatomy, and the old lady said, "I don't want to know it. Just do it!"

Was this Bennett the Touretter being obsessive or Professor Bennett the lecturer on anatomy? (He gives weekly anatomy lectures in Calgary.) Was it simply an expression of his meticulousness and concern? An imagining, perhaps, that all patients shared his curiosity and love of detail? Some patients doubtless did, but obviously not these.

So it went on through a lengthy outpatient list. Bennett is evidently a very popular surgeon, and he saw or operated on each patient swiftly and dexterously, with an absolute and single-minded concentration, so that when they saw him they knew they had his whole attention. They forgot that they had waited, or that there were others still waiting, and felt that for him they were the only people in the world.

Very pleasant, very real, the surgeon's life, I kept thinking—direct, friendly relationships, especially clear with outpatients like this. An immediacy of relation, of work, of results, of gratification—much greater than with a physician, especially a neurologist (like me). I thought of my mother, how much she enjoyed the surgeon's life, and how I always loved sitting in at her surgical outpatient rounds. I could not become a surgeon myself, because of an incorrigible clumsiness, but even as a child I had loved the surgeon's life, and watching surgeons at work. This love, this pleasure, half forgotten, came back to me with great force as I observed Bennett with his patients; made me want to be more than a spectator; made me want to do something, to hold a retractor, to join in somehow in the surgery.

Bennett's last patient was a young mechanic with extensive neurofibromatosis, a bizarre and sometimes cancerous disease that can produce huge brownish swellings and protruding sheets of skin, disfiguring the whole body. This young man had had a huge apron of tissue hanging down from his chest, so large that he could lift it up and cover his head, and so heavy that it bowed him forward with its weight. Bennett had removed this a couple of weeks earlier—a massive procedure—with great expertise and was now examining another huge apron descending from the shoulders, and great flaps of brownish flesh in the groins and armpits. I was relieved that he did not tic "Hideous!" as he removed the stitches from the surgery, for I feared the impact of such a word being uttered aloud, even if it was nothing but a long-standing verbal tic. But, mercifully, there was no "Hideous," there were no verbal tics at all, until Bennett was examining the dorsal skin flap and let fly a brief "Hid——," the end of the word omitted by a tactful apocope. This, I learned later, was not a conscious suppression—Bennett had no memory of the tic—and yet it seemed to me there must have been, if not a conscious, then a subconscious solicitude and tact at work. "Fine young man," Bennett said, as we went outside. "Not self-conscious. Nice personality, outgoing. Most people with this would lock themselves in a closet." I could not help feeling that his words could also be applied to himself. There are many people with Tourette's who become agonized and self-conscious, withdraw from the world, and lock themselves in a closet. Not so Bennett: he had struggled against this; he had come through and braved life, braved people, braved the most improbable of professions. All his patients, I think, perceived this, and it was one of the reasons they trusted him so.

The man with the skin flap was the last of the outpatients, but for Bennett, immensely busy, there was only a brief break before an equally long afternoon with his inpatients on the ward. I excused myself from this to take an afternoon off and walk around the town. I wandered through Branford with the oddest sense of déjà vu and *jamais vu* mixed; I kept feeling that I had seen the town before, but then again that it was new to me. And then, suddenly, I had it—yes, I had seen it, I had been here before, for a night in August 1960, when it had a population of only a few thousand and consisted of little more than a few dusty streets, motels, bars—a crossroads, little more than a truck stop in the long trek across the west. Now its population was twenty thousand, Main Street a gleaming boulevard filled with shops and cars; there was a town hall, a police station, a regional hospital, several schools—it was this that surrounded me, the overwhelming present, yet through it I saw the dusty crossroads and the bars, the Branford of thirty years before, still strangely vivid, because never updated, in my mind.

Friday is operating day for Bennett, and he was scheduled to do a mastectomy. I was eager to join him, to see him in action. Outpatients are one thing—one can always concentrate for a few minutes—but how would he conduct himself in a lengthy and difficult procedure demanding intense, unremitting concentration, not for seconds or minutes but for hours?

Bennett preparing for the operating room was a startling sight.

"You should scrub next to him," his young assistant said. "It's quite an experience." It was indeed, for what I saw in the outpatient clinic was magnified here: constant sudden dartings and reachings with the hands, almost but never quite touching his unscrubbed, unsterile shoulder, his assistant, the mirror; sudden lungings and touchings of his colleagues with his feet; and a barrage of vocalizations—"Hooty-hooo! Hooty-hooo!"—suggestive of a huge owl.

The scrubbing over, Bennett and his assistant were gloved and gowned, and they moved to the patient, already anesthetized, on the table. They looked briefly at a mammogram on the X-ray box. Then Bennett took the knife, made a bold, clear incision—there was no hint of any ticcing or distraction—and moved straightaway into the rhythm of the operation. Twenty minutes passed, fifty, seventy, a hundred. The operation was often complex—vessels to be tied, nerves to be found—but the action was confident, smooth, moving forward at its own pace, with never the slightest hint of Tourette's. Finally, after two and a half hours of the most complex, taxing surgery, Bennett closed up, thanked everybody, yawned, and stretched. Here, then, was an entire operation without a trace of Tourette's. Not because it had been suppressed, or held in—there was never any sign of control or constraint—but because, simply, there was never any impulse to tic. "Most of the time when I'm operating, it never even crosses my mind that I have Tourette's," Bennett says. His whole identity at such times is that of a surgeon at work, and his entire psychic and neural organization becomes aligned with this, becomes active, focused, at ease, un-Tourettic. It is only if the operation is broken for a few minutes—to review a special X ray taken during the surgery, for example—that Bennett, waiting, unoccupied, remembers that he *is* Tourettic, and in that instant he becomes so. As soon as the flow of the operation resumes, the Tourette's, the Tourettic identity, vanishes once again. Bennett's assistants, though they have known him and worked with him for years, are still astounded whenever they see this. "It's like a miracle," one of them says. "The way the Tourette's disappears." And Bennett himself is astonished, too, and quizzes me, as he peels off his gloves, on the neurophysiology of it all.

Things were not always so easy, Bennett told me later. Occasionally, if he was bombarded by outside demands during surgery— "You have three patients waiting in the ER," "Mrs. X wants to know if she can come in on the tenth," "Your wife wants you to pick up three bags of dog food"—these pressures, these distractions, would break his concentration, break the smooth and rhythmic flow. A couple of years ago, he made it a rule that he must never be disturbed while operating and must be allowed to concentrate totally on the surgery, and the OR has been tic-free ever since.

Friday afternoon is open. Bennett often likes to go for long hikes on Fridays, or cycle rides, or drives, with a sense of the trail, the open road, before him. There is a favorite ranch he loves to go to, with a beautiful lake and an airstrip, accessible only via a rugged dirt road. It is a wonderfully situated ranch, a narrow fertile strip perfectly placed between the lake and mountains, and we walked for miles, talking of this and that, with Bennett botanizing or geologizing as we went. Then, briefly, we went to the lake, where I took a swim; when I came out of the water I found that Bennett, rather suddenly, had curled up for a nap. He looked peaceful, tension free, as he slept; and the suddenness and depth of his sleep made me wonder how much difficulty he encountered in the daytime, how much he concealed beneath his genial surface—how much, inwardly, he had to control and deal with.

Later, as we continued our ramble about the ranch, he remarked that I had seen only some of the outward expressions of his Tourette's, and these, bizarre as they occasionally seemed, were by no means the worst problems it caused him. The real problems, the inner problems, were panic and rage—feelings so violent that they threatened to overwhelm him, and so sudden that he had virtually no warning of their onset. He had only to get a parking ticket or see a police car, sometimes, for scenarios of violence to flash through his mind: mad chases, shoot-outs, flaming destruction, hideous mutilation and death—scenarios that would become immensely elaborated in seconds and rush through his mind with manic Tourettic speed. One part of him, uninvolved, could watch these scenes with detachment, but another part of him was taken over and felt impelled to action. He could prevent himself from giving way to outbursts in public, but the strain of controlling himself was severe and exhausting. At home, in private, he could let himself go—not at others but at inanimate objects around him. There was the wall I had seen, which he had often struck in his rage, and the refrigerator, at which he had flung virtually everything in the kitchen. In his office, he had kicked a hole in the wall and had had to put a plant in front of it to cover it; and in his study at home the cedar walls were covered with knife marks. "It's not gentle," he said to me. "You can see it as whimsical, funny—be tempted to romanticize it—but Tourette's comes from deep down in the nervous system and the unconscious. It taps into the oldest, strongest feelings we have. Tourette's is like an epilepsy in the subcortex; when it takes over, there's just a thin line of control, a thin line of cortex, between you and it, between you and that raging storm, the blind force of the subcortex. One can see the charming things, the funny things, the creative side of Tourette's, but there's also that dark side. You have to fight it all your life."

Driving back from the ranch was a stimulating, at times terrifying, experience. Now that Bennett was getting to know me, he felt at liberty to let himself and his Tourette's go. The steering wheel was abandoned for seconds at a time—or so it seemed to me, in my alarm—while he tapped on the windshield (to a litany of "Hootyhoo!" and "Hi, there!" and "Hideous!"), rearranged his glasses, "centered" them in a hundred different ways, and, with bent forefingers, continually smoothed and evened his mustache while gazing in the rearview mirror rather than at the road. His need to center the steering wheel in relation to his knees also grew almost frenetic at this time: he had constantly to "balance" it, to jerk it to and fro, causing the car to zigzag erratically down the road. "Don't worry," he said when he saw my anxiety. "I know this road. I could see from way back that nothing was coming. I've never had an accident driving."

The impulse to look, and to be looked at, is very striking with Bennett, and, indeed, as soon as we got back to the house, he seized Mark and planted himself in front of him, smoothing his mustache furiously and saying, "Look at me! Look at me!" Mark, arrested, stayed where he was, but his eyes wandered to and fro. Now Bennett seized Mark's head, held it rigidly toward him, hissing, "Look, look at me!" And Mark became totally still, transfixed, as if hypnotized.

I found this scene disquieting. Other scenes with the family I had found rather moving: Bennett dabbing at Helen's hair, symmetrically, with outstretched fingers, going "whoo, whoo" softly. She was placid, accepting; it was a touching scene, both tender and absurd. "I love him as he is," Helen said. "I wouldn't want him any other way." Bennett feels the same way: "Funny disease—I don't think of it as a disease but as just me. I say the word 'disease,' but it doesn't seem to be the appropriate word."

Though Bennett is quite prepared, even eager, to think of Tourette's in neurochemical or neurophysiological terms—he thinks in terms of chemical abnormalities, of "circuits turning on and off," and of "primitive, normally inhibited behaviors being released"— he also feels it as something that has come to be part of himself. For this reason (among others), he has found that he cannot tolerate haloperidol and similar drugs—they reduce his Tourette's, assuredly, but they reduce *him* as well, so that he no longer feels fully himself. "The side effects of haloperidol were dreadful," he said. "I was intensely restless, I couldn't stand still, my body twisted, I shuffled like a Parkinsonian. It was a huge relief to get off it. On the other hand, Prozac has been a godsend for the obsessions, the rages, though it doesn't touch the tics." Prozac has indeed been a godsend for many Touretters, though some have found it to have no effect, and a few have had paradoxical effects—an intensification of their agitations, obsessions, and rages.

Though Bennett has had tics since the age of seven or so, he did not identify what he had as Tourette's syndrome until he was thirty-seven. "When we were first married, he just called it a nervous habit," Helen told me. "We used to joke about it. I'd say, 'I'll quit smoking, and you quit twitching.' We thought of it as something he *could* quit if he wanted. You'd ask him, 'Why do you do it?' He'd say, 'I don't know why.' He didn't seem to be self-conscious about it. Then, in 1977, when Mark was a baby, Carl heard this program, 'Quirks and Quarks,' on the radio. He got all excited and hollered, 'Helen, come listen! This guy's talking about what I do!' He was excited to hear that other people had it. And it was a relief to me, because I had always sensed that there was something wrong. It was good to put a label on it. He never made a thing of it, he wouldn't raise the subject, but once we knew, we'd tell people if they asked. It's only in the last few years that he's met other people with it, or gone to meetings of the Tourette Syndrome Association [TSA]." (Tourette's syndrome, until very recently, was remarkably under-diagnosed and unknown, even to the medical profession, and most people diagnosed themselves, or were diagnosed by friends and family, after seeing or reading something about it in the media. Indeed, I know of another doctor, a surgeon in Louisiana, who was diagnosed by one of his own patients who had seen a Touretter on *Donahue*. Much of this media emphasis has been due to the efforts of the TSA, which had only thirty members in the early seventies but now has more than twenty thousand.)

Saturday morning, and I have to return to New York. "I'll fly you to Calgary if the weather's fine," Bennett said suddenly last night. "Ever flown with a Touretter before?"

I had canoed with one, I said, and driven across country with another, but flying with one . . .

"You'll enjoy it," Bennett said. "It'll be a novel experience. I am the world's only flying Touretter surgeon."

When I awake, at dawn, I perceive, with mixed feelings, that the weather, though very cold, is perfect. We drive to the little airport in Branford, a veering, twitching journey that makes me nervous about the flight. "It's much easier in the air, where there's no road to keep to, and you don't have to keep your hands on the controls all the time," Bennett says. At the airport, he parks, opens a hangar, and proudly points out his airplane—a tiny red-and-white single-engine Cessna Cardinal. He pulls it out onto the tarmac and then checks it, rechecks it, and re-rechecks it before warming up the engine. It is near freezing on the airfield, and a north wind is blowing. I watch all the checks and rechecks with impatience but also with a sense of reassurance. If his Tourette's makes him check everything three or five times, so much the safer. I had a similar feeling of reassurance about his surgery—that his Tourette's, if anything, made him more meticulous, more exact, without in the least damping down his intuitiveness, his freedom.

His checking done, Bennett leaps like a trapeze artist into the plane, revs the engine while I climb in, and takes off. As we climb, the sun is rising over the Rockies to the east, and floods the little cabin with a pale, golden light. We head toward nine-thousand-foot crests, and Bennett tics, flutters, reaches, taps, touches his glasses, his mustache, the top of the cockpit. Minor tics, Little League, I think, but what if he has big tics? What if he wants to twirl the plane in midair, to hop and skip with it, to do somersaults, to loop the loop? What if he has an impulse to leap out and touch the propeller? Touretters tend to be fascinated by spinning objects; I have a vision of him lunging forward, half out the window, compulsively lunging at the propeller before us. But his tics and compulsions remain very minor, and when he takes his hands off the controls the plane continues quietly. Mercifully, there is no road to keep to. If we rise or fall or veer fifty feet, what does it matter? We have the whole sky to play with.

And Bennett, though superbly skilled, a natural aviator, *is* like a child at play. Part of Tourette's, at least, is no more than this—the release of a playful impulse normally inhibited or lost in the rest of us. The freedom, the spaciousness obviously delight Bennett; he has a carefree, boyish look I rarely saw on the ground. Now, rising, we fly over the first peaks, the advance guard of the Rockies; yellowing larches stream beneath us. We clear the slopes by a thousand feet or more. I wonder whether Bennett, if he were by himself, might want to clear the peaks by ten feet, by inches—Touretters are sometimes addicted to close shaves. At ten thousand feet, we move in a corridor between peaks, mountains shining in the morning sun to our left, mountains silhouetted against it to our right. At eleven thousand feet, we can see the whole width of the Rockies—they are only fifty-five miles across here—and the vast golden Alberta prairie starting to the east. Every so often, Bennett's right hand flutters in front of me, or his hand taps lightly on the windshield. "Sedimentary rocks, look!" He gestures through the window. "Lifted up from the sea bottom at seventy to eighty degrees." He gazes at the steeply sloping rocks as at a friend; he is intensely at home with these mountains, this land. Snow lies on the sunless slopes of the mountains, none yet on their sunlit faces; and over to the northwest, toward Banff, we can see glaciers on the mountains. Bennett shifts, and shifts, and shifts again, trying to get his knees exactly symmetrical beneath the controls of the plane.

In Alberta now—we have been flying for forty minutes—the Highwood River winds beneath us. Flying due north, we start a gentle descent toward Calgary, the last, declining slopes of the Rockies all shimmering with aspen. Now, lower, to vast fields of wheat and alfalfa—farms, ranches, fertile prairie—but still, everywhere, stands of golden aspen. Beyond the checkerboard of fields, the towers of Calgary rise abruptly from the flat plain.

Suddenly, the radio crackles alive—a giant Russian air transport is coming in; the main runway, closed for maintenance, must quickly be opened up. And another massive plane, from the Zambian Air Force. The world's planes come to Calgary for special work and maintenance; its facilities, Bennett tells me, are some of the best in North America. In the middle of this important flurry, Bennett radios in our position and statistics (fifteen-foot-long Cardinal, with a Touretter and his neurologist) and is immediately answered, as fully and helpfully as if he were a 747. All planes, all pilots are equal in this world. And it is a world apart, with a freemasonry of its own, its own language, codes, myths, and manners. Bennett, clearly, is part of this world, and is recognized by the traffic controller and greeted cheerfully as he taxis in.

He leaps out with a startling, ticlike suddenness and celerity—I follow at a slower, "normal" pace—and starts talking with two giant young men on the tarmac, Kevin and Chuck, brothers, both fourth-generation pilots in the Rockies. They know him well. "He's just one of us," Chuck says to me. "A regular guy. Tourette's—what the hell? He's a good human being. A damn good pilot, too."

Bennett yarns with his fellow pilots and files his flight plan for the return trip to Branford. He has to return straightaway; he is due to speak at eleven to a group of nurses, and his subject, for once, is not surgery but Tourette's. His little plane is refueled and readied for the return flight. We hug and say good-bye, and as I head for my flight to New York, I turn to watch him go. Bennett walks to his plane, taxis onto the main runway, and takes off, fast, with a tail wind following. I watch him for a while, and then he is gone.

lee gutkind

Creative nonfiction writers will often immerse themselves, on the scene, and wait for something totally spontaneous to happen—a moment that signals the direction of the narrative and solidifies meaning and/or focus. In this chapter from *An Unspoken Art,* two defining moments occur: (1) when Jason enters the operating room, and (2) when Solomon reveals to Jason a secret that helps facilitate a mutual acceptance and understanding of grief and recovery.

an unspoken art

Working swiftly, Dr. Gene Solomon, a blue paper hat and mask concealing his head and face, quickly gowns, soaps, scrubs, and dries his hands, snaps on a pair of surgical gloves, arranges a set of blue towels around the surgical field, lifts a scalpel—and cuts. A couple of flicks of the wrist, and he's suddenly groping around, elbow deep inside the poodle's abdominal area, as if reaching for a glove or cap stuffed into a coat sleeve.

"This dog came in two days ago. Swallowed a sock." Solomon had waited to see if the dog passed the sock or parts of the sock in its stool before taking action. "But the dog was getting sick. He couldn't pee. His spleen was inflamed. An emergency exploration was required. "'Foreign bodies' often cause serious problems," Solomon said. It will take at least another half hour to locate and meticulously remove the remainder of the sock and sew the dog back up again. Foreign-body surgery, often time consuming and challenging, is a routine part of domestic veterinary practice.

"Close your eyes and imagine," Solomon tells me. "'Foreign body' possibilities are limitless. Cassette tape, rubber balls, tennis balls, lingerie, jewelry, elastic strips, fan belts, and once, a set of eyeglasses—this from the littlest dog you've ever seen with the biggest mouth imaginable." And coins; pennies made before 1982, which were 97 percent copper, are less harmful than pennies after that date because the composition changed; they became 97 percent zinc. And zinc destroys red blood cells, thus causing the animal to become extremely anemic, a life-threatening condition.

Cats are the most difficult foreign-body cases. Strings seem harmless, but Solomon was once confronted with a cat that was bleeding to death because a string had gotten wrapped around the intestinal tract, shrunk, and sliced the bowel in half. Solomon removed thirty inches of bowel and saved the cat's life. During the Christmas holidays, it is very popular for cats to swallow tinsel. "I actually met one of my fiancées through foreign-body surgery. Her dog swallowed a rubber toy, and she came to our hospital, panicked. I calmed her down."

Solomon, thirty-nine, has never been married, but is no stranger to entanglements and engagements. Like medical doctors, police officers, and others involved in all-consuming professions, Solomon is obsessed by his work. "My mother said that from the time I was five years old, I was bringing animals home and trying to take care of them." He offers a flourishing gesture with a feces-caked clamp, forcing everyone in the room to flinch or duck their heads. "Today, I do house calls all over the world: Florida, California, Jamaica. Clients that I've met over the years, some of whom have moved away, would rather fly me down to wherever they are than get a new doctor. Some of the wealthiest people in the world. I mean, *in the world,*" Solomon says. "I have a client who just left yesterday to go to Paris on the Concorde with her dog. The dog sits on the seat next to her, the two of them together."

A need to know often distinguishes the Manhattan resident from most other clients. When people say, "What do you think caused my dog to get this condition?" the New York veterinarian is usually given permission to do diagnostic tests, skin scraping, blood tests, X rays, biopsies, tests that may be informative, but not cost effective. "People in the suburbs say to their doctors, 'Look, what made my dog get sick?' And the veterinarian says, 'Well, if you want to find out, it will cost you a hundred and fifty dollars.' And they say, 'That's too much. Fix the dog. I don't need to know why it happened.'

"But Manhattan has a great number of people without children, a great number of people who are by themselves. The animals become members of the family. As a result, you get two people who are living together; they have two incomes; they have no kids; they have no tuitions; they are consequently able to give the animal the kind of care that a typical suburban family, who can't afford to go the full nine yards, won't." On the Upper East Side, veterinarians will seldom euthanize animals because owners can't afford to care for them, a more common occurrence elsewhere.

As Gene Solomon continued his painstaking task of removing the swallowed sock, thread by thread and inch by inch, he explained that cats, from an anatomical and physiological point of view, were wholly unique. "One Tylenol in a cat is a good way to put them to sleep forever, whereas in a dog, Tylenol is not as damaging." Cats lack the liver enzymes to metabolize Tylenol correctly. For those cats who do metabolize it, Tylenol becomes an oxidizing agent. "Their blood turns brown. Their membranes turn brown. A cat can die from just one Tylenol within twenty-four hours without treatment." Cats also hide disease better than dogs.

Concealing pain and sickness is part of the natural instinct to live life with bravado, as a first line of defense against natural enemies. Animals are also unable to communicate physical deterioration. By the time such an easily treatable problem as glaucoma is diagnosed, for example, an animal may be blind in one eye. Dogs and cats cannot tell their owners that they have a headache or cannot see. Animals may experience pain and sickness in the same manner as people do, but they accept such discomfort and inconvenience as a way of life. In most veterinary emergency centers, trauma—auto accidents, dog fights, cats jumping out of high-rises—is most prevalent, as well as toxins, rat poison, and antifreeze.

Understanding animal anatomy is perhaps the most awesome and ongoing task for a veterinarian—and a primary way in which to distinguish the challenges and complications of human and animal medicine. The human is probably the most sophisticated animal, but humans are also miraculously and consistently similar despite age, race, and nationality. Cats, dogs, birds, and the like are entirely different, physiologically and anatomically. Each animal presents a unique anatomical challenge.

Some veterinarians, especially those in rural areas, will treat any species that cross the threshold of their office or hospital. Solomon and Schwartz have chosen to narrow the range of the species they are willing to treat to dogs and cats and other domestics to which clients in this prosperous neighborhood take a fancy. Although they are basically general practice, occasionally Schwartz will perform acupuncture, while Solomon is known for his work in oncology.

"Yesterday," said Solomon, "I put to sleep a patient who has been with me for three years. It was my hardest and most difficult case, ever. The owner, Pauline Wilson, was committed and obsessed. She was on the phone to me, literally, in the three years since we first met, at least once a day. No matter where I was in the world, she talked to me, sometimes half a dozen, sometimes a dozen times a day. Her cat had cancer of the jaw. I operated, removed the jaw. Cured the cancer. That was two years ago. But from that point onward, the animal had to be fed by hand. Pauline and her husband were willing to do this four times a day, day after day, for two years. And if that animal missed a meal or was off a little bit, they were on the phone, hysterical. This animal could not really walk around very well, but you see, the cat was happy. It watched television and looked out the window, and the family was comfortable with that."

"But *you* weren't comfortable," one of the veterinary technicians assisting with the surgery interjected.

"But it doesn't matter if I'm comfortable, subjectively speaking," says Solomon. "I only had to be comfortable objectively. Do you follow? 'Subjectively' means emotion . . . how I feel about it personally. Which has nothing to do with what is right or wrong. Objectively, I knew that animal was not suffering. Objectively I knew that animal was not in pain, so I was fulfilling my responsibility as a veterinarian to the owner and the animal, and I could live very easily with that."

"How much money did Pauline invest over the three-year period in which you were treating the cat?" I asked.

"Enormous amounts," Solomon replied. "She could spend five hundred dollars a week in here. Easily. Listen," he shrugged and continued, "I have many clients like that. I am always honest with them. I'll say, 'To get your animal from here to there, say six months of life, will cost ten thousand dollars,' something like that. People will go for it. Money is not an issue in this practice. Pauline loved her cat—lived for her cat; she refused to give up on her cat. Many people don't understand the deep level of emotion that the loss of an animal can cause a human being, but after so many years of being together, losing a pet can be like losing a spouse or a child—or sometimes worse." Pauline invested more than $50,000 over a three-year period to keep her beloved Baby Cat alive.

Just then, as if on cue, a neatly groomed, nattily dressed man in his early forties pressed his nose against the window and asked Solomon through an abbreviated set of hand signals if he could enter. Solomon nodded and the man disappeared, then quickly reappeared, awkwardly arranging a blue mask and cap and easing himself into Solomon's surgical inner sanctum. "How are you doing today, Jason?" Although Solomon can be hard edged, wisecracking, and cynical, his tone and manner visibly softened when Jason entered the room.

"I'm doing okay, Gene," Jason replied. "Better than yesterday." Jason paused and swallowed. He lowered his head. Suddenly, without warning, he began to sob. "Gene," he choked, "Beau. It's been a week and a day since he died."

Solomon continued to remove pieces of feces-caked sock from the dog's small intestine. "This has been a very hard time for you, Jason, but it's understandable not to be dealing so well. You and Beau were together eight years. If this was easy—for any of us—then we wouldn't have been so invested in our animals. The burden of our grief signifies the greatness of our loss."

Once again, Jason dabs his eyes and blows his nose. "I really am sorry," he says to no one in particular.

"There's nothing to be sorry about, Jason," Solomon assures him, as he neatly and nimbly completes the process of stitching his patient. In Manhattan, "cosmetics" are priority. Owners are very sensitive as to how much hair is shaved prior to the surgery, as well as the extent and predominance of the scar after the surgery is completed. Finally feeling satisfied with his work, Solomon backs away from the table. He pulls off his gloves and tosses them into a nearby wastebasket, motioning to Jason to follow him. Fifteen minutes later, Jason appears once more. Again, he has been crying; his red face glistens with tears. But he is also calmer and he is clutching a small corrugated cardboard box tightly to his chest as he leaves the hospital.

Later, Solomon is sitting in the cluttered office he shares with his partner, his hiking boots propped on his desk, while he wolfs down a roast beef sandwich and chugs a two-liter bottle of Pepsi. At first glance, Gene Solomon looks completely unlike any veterinarian one would imagine. He's young; his black hair is swept back; his teeth are widely spaced. He talks fast and walks fast; his style and mannerisms are much more reminiscent of a Manhattan attorney than a veterinarian. He is talking about Jason.

"At first, he was kind of a distant friend I would see once in a while, socially, but we became much closer last year when I began giving his dog chemotherapy. Beau was a great dog and a brave dog. The morning of his death, Beau played for a few minutes in the park. It was a bittersweet ending."

That day, after Beau and Jason returned home from the park, Solomon canceled his late afternoon appointments and walked to Jason's apartment. In the living room, they talked quietly, Solomon all the while assuring Jason that he was doing the right thing, the only thing he could do for the dog and faithful friend whom he loved, considering the circumstances. Now Jason removed the bottle of champagne that had been chilling in the ice bucket on the coffee table, popped the cork, and poured two brimming glasses. They lifted their glasses slowly, and both men, owner and doctor, toasted their friend Beau in a very special and personal way. Then Gene quickly took the hypodermic needle that he had readied the moment he arrived and quickly and quietly injected Beau with sodium phenobarbital. Beau shuddered just once and settled for one last moment of togetherness in Jason's lap. He died quickly.

"Jason was here today to pick up Beau's ashes," Solomon tells me between bites of his sandwich and phone messages related by the office manager over the intercom. "He was feeling quite vulnerable. That's one reason he was so emotional in the operating room. This is the final part—and he feels foolish for wanting to keep the ashes with him at home. He told me: 'People will think it is weird.'"

"And what did you tell him?" I said.

He shrugged. "There wasn't much to say," Solomon replied. He chewed thoughtfully, then leaned forward, wiping his hands nervously on his black Levis and smiling sheepishly. "Well, you saw where we went." He pointed out the door in the direction of the corridor in which he and Jason had disappeared. "There's a cabinet back there where I keep a few important personal possessions, and that's where I took him."

Solomon had opened the door of the cabinet for Jason, reached up to the top shelf, and proceeded to pull out a leash and a collar and a jar of ashes from a dog he had euthanized. "This was my dog," he told Jason. "She died a little less than two years ago, but I keep these ashes close to where I spend most of my time. So, Jason, I guess I am just as weird as you."

leonard kriegel

The image of falling is the glue that binds this moving and inspiring essay. The title—"Falling into Life"—represents what the reader learns about recovery from, or rehabilitation with polio. But Kriegel makes many additional thematic connections: "Falling from physical grace" is what happens when you actually get polio, as is falling away from "the body's prowess." Falling into life is not a metaphor—but a real necessity, as is "falling into death," which he hopes to experience as "nakedly as I once had to fall into life."

falling into life

It is not the actual death a man is doomed to die but the deaths his imagination anticipates that claim attention as one grows older. We are constantly being reminded that the prospect of death forcefully concentrates the mind. While that may be so, it is not a prospect that does very much else for the imagination—other than to make one aware of its limitations and imbalances.

Over the past five years, as I have moved into the solidity of middle age, my own most formidable imaginative limitation has turned out to be a surprising need for symmetry. I am possessed by a peculiar passion: I want to believe that my life has been balanced out. And because I once had to learn to fall in order to keep that life mine, I now seem to have convinced myself that I must also learn to fall into death.

Falling into life wasn't easy, and I suspect that is why I hunger for such awkward symmetry today. Having lost the use of my legs during the polio epidemic that swept across the eastern United States during the summer of 1944, I was soon immersed in a process of rehabilitation that was, at least when looked at in retrospect, as much spiritual as physical.

That was a full decade before the discovery of the Salk vaccine ended polio's reign as the disease most dreaded by America's parents and their children. Treatment of the disease had been standardized by 1944: following the initial onslaught of the virus, patients were kept in isolation for a period of ten days to two weeks. Following that, orthodox medical opinion was content to subject patients to as much heat as they could stand. Stiff paralyzed limbs were swathed in heated, coarse woolen towels known as "hot packs." (The towels were that same greenish brown as blankets issued to American GIs, and they reinforced a boy's sense of being at war.) As soon as the hot packs had baked enough pain and stiffness out of a patient's body so that he could be moved on and off a stretcher, the treatment was ended, and the patient faced a series of daily immersions in a heated pool.

I would ultimately spend two full years at the appropriately named New York State Reconstruction Home in West Haverstraw. But what I remember most vividly about the first three months of my stay there was being submerged in a hot pool six times a day, for periods of between fifteen and twenty minutes. I would lie on a stainless steel slab, my face alone out of water, while the wet heat rolled against my dead legs and the physical therapist was at my side working at a series of manipulations intended to bring my useless muscles back to health.

Each immersion was a baptism by fire in the water. While my mind pitched and reeled with memories of the "normal" boy I had been a few weeks earlier, I would close my eyes and focus not, as my therapist urged, on bringing dead legs back to life but on my strange fall from the childhood grace of the physical. Like all eleven-year-old boys, I had spent a good deal of time thinking about my body. Before the attack of the virus, however, I thought about it only in connection with my own lunge toward adolescence. Never before had my body seemed an object in itself. Now it was. And like the twenty-one other boys in the ward—all of us between the ages of nine and twelve—I sensed I would never move beyond the fall from grace, even as I played with memories of the way I once had been.

Each time I was removed from the hot water and placed on a stretcher by the side of the pool, there to await the next immersion, I was fed salt tablets. These were simply intended to make up for the sweat we lost, but salt tablets seemed to me the cruelest confirmation of my new status as spiritual debtor. Even today, more than four decades later, I still shiver at the mere thought of those salt tablets. Sometimes the hospital orderly would literally have to pry my mouth open to force me to swallow them. I dreaded the nausea the taste of salt inspired in me. Each time I was resubmerged in the hot pool, I would grit my teeth—not from the flush of heat sweeping over my body but from the thought of what I would have to face when I would again be taken out of the water. To be an eater of salt was far more humiliating than to endure pain. Nor was I alone in feeling this way. After lights-out had quieted the ward, we boys would furtively whisper from cubicle to cubicle of how we dreaded being forced to swallow salt tablets. It was that, rather than the pain we endured, that anchored our sense of loss and dread.

Any recovery of muscle use in a polio patient usually took place within three months of the disease's onset. We all knew that. But as time passed, every boy in the ward learned to recite stories of those who, like Lazarus, had witnessed their own bodily resurrection. Having fallen from physical grace, we also chose to fall away from the reality in front of us. Our therapists were skilled and dedicated, but they weren't wonder-working saints. Paralyzed legs and arms rarely responded to their manipulations. We could not admit to ourselves, or to them, that we were permanently crippled. But each of us knew without knowing that his future was tied to the body that floated on the stainless steel slab.

We sweated out the hot pool and we choked on the salt tablets, and through it all we looked forward to the promise of rehabilitation. For, once the stiffness and pain had been baked and boiled out of us, we would no longer be eaters of salt. We would not be what we once had been, but at least we would be candidates for reentry into the world, admittedly made over to face its demands encased in leather and steel.

I suppose we might have been told that our fall from grace was permanent. But I am still grateful that no one—neither doctors nor nurses nor therapists, not even that sadistic orderly, himself a former polio patient, who limped through our lives and through our pain like some vengeful presence—told me that my chances of regaining the use of my legs were nonexistent. Like every other boy in the ward, I organized my needs around whatever illusions were available. And the illusion I needed above any other was that one morning I would simply wake up and rediscover the "normal" boy of memory, once again playing baseball in French Charley's Field in Bronx Park rather than roaming the fields of his own imagination. At the age of eleven, I needed to weather reality, not face it. And to this very day, I silently thank those who were concerned enough about me, or indifferent enough to my fate, not to tell me what they knew.

Like most boys, sick or well, I was an adaptable creature—and rehabilitation demanded adaptability. The fall from bodily grace transformed each of us into acolytes of the possible, pragmatic Americans for whom survival was method and strategy. We would learn, during our days in the New York State Reconstruction Home, to confront the world that was. We would learn to survive the way we were, with whatever the virus had left intact.

I had fallen away from the body's prowess, but I was being led toward a life measured by different standards. Even as I fantasized about the past, it disappeared. Rehabilitation, I was to learn, was ahistorical, a future devoid of any significant claim on the past. Rehabilitation was a thief's primer of compensation and deception: its purpose was to teach one how to steal a touch of the normal from an existence that would be striking in its abnormality.

When I think back to those two years in the ward, the boy who made his rehabilitation most memorable was Joey Tomashevski. Joey was the son of an upstate dairy farmer, a Polish immigrant who had come to America before the depression and whose English was even poorer than the English of my own shtetl-bred father. The virus had left both of Joey's arms so lifeless and atrophied that I could circle where his bicep should have been with pinky and thumb and still stick the forefinger of my own hand through. And yet, Joey assumed that he would make do with whatever had been left him. He accepted without question the task of making his toes and feet over into fingers and hands. With lifeless arms encased in a canvas sling that looked like the breadbasket a European peasant might carry to market, Joey would sit up in bed and demonstrate how he could maneuver fork and spoon with his toes.

I would never have dreamed of placing such confidence in my fingers, let alone my toes. I found, as most of the other boys in the ward did, Joey's unabashed pride in the flexibility and control with which he could maneuver a forkful of mashed potatoes into his mouth a continuous indictment of my sense of the world's natural order. We boys with dead legs would gather round his bed in our wheelchairs and silently watch Joey display his dexterity with a vanity so open and naked that it seemed an invitation to being struck down yet again. But Joey's was a vanity already tested by experience. For he was more than willing to accept whatever challenges the virus threw his way. For the sake of demonstrating his skill to us, he kicked a basketball from the auditorium stage through the hoop attached to a balcony some fifty feet away. When one of our number derisively called him lucky, he proceeded to kick five of seven more balls through that same hoop.

I suspect that Joey's pride in his ability to compensate for what had been taken away from him irritated me, because I knew that before I could pursue my own rehabilitation with such singular passion, I had to surrender myself to what was being demanded of me. And that meant I had to learn to fall. It meant that I had to learn, as Joey Tomashevski had already learned, how to transform absence into opportunity. Even though I still lacked Joey's instinctive willingness to live with the legacy of the virus, I found myself being overhauled, re-created in much the same way as a car engine is rebuilt. Nine months after I arrived in the ward, a few weeks before my twelfth birthday, I was fitted for double long-legged braces bound together by a steel pelvic band circling my waist. Lifeless or not, my legs were precisely measured, the steel carefully molded to form, screws and locks and leather joined to one another for my customized benefit alone. It was technology that would hold me up—another offering on the altar of compensation. "You get what you give," said Jackie Lyons, my closest friend in the ward. He, too, now had to learn how to choose the road back.

Falling into life was not a metaphor; it was real, a process learned only through doing, the way a baby learns to crawl, to stand, and then to walk. After the steel bands around calves and thighs and pelvis had been covered over by the rich-smelling leather, after the braces had been precisely fitted to allow my fear-ridden imagination the surety of their holding presence, I was pulled to my feet. For the first time in ten months, I stood. Two middle-aged craftsmen, the hospital bracemakers who worked in a machine shop deep in the basement, held me in place as my therapist wedged two wooden crutches beneath my shoulders.

They stepped back, first making certain that my grip on the crutches was firm. Filled with pride in their technological prowess, the three of them stood in front of me, admiring their skill. Had I been created in the laboratory of Mary Shelley's Dr. Frankenstein, I could not have felt myself any more the creature of scientific pride. I stood on the braces, crutches beneath my shoulders slanting outward like twin towers of Pisa. I flushed, swallowed hard, struggled to keep from crying, struggled not to be overwhelmed by my fear of falling.

My future had arrived. The leather had been fitted, the screws had been turned to the precise millimeter, the locks at the knees and the bushings at the ankles had been properly tested and retested. That very afternoon I was taken for the first time to a cavernous room filled with barbells and Indian clubs and crutches and walkers. I would spend an hour each day there for the next six months. In the rehab room, I would learn how to mount two large wooden steps made to the exact measure of those of a New York City bus. I would swing on parallel bars from one side to the other, my arms learning how they would have to hurl me through the world. I balanced Indian clubs like a circus juggler because my therapist insisted it would help my coordination. And I was expected to learn to fall.

I was a dutiful patient. I did as I was told because I could see no advantage to doing anything else. I hungered for the approval of those in authority—doctors, nurses, therapists, the two bracemakers. Again and again, my therapist demonstrated how I was to throw my legs from the hip. Again and again, I did as I was told. Grabbing the banister with my left hand, I threw my leg from the hip while pushing off my right crutch. Like some baby elephant (despite the sweat lost in the heated pool, the months of inactivity in bed had fattened me up considerably), I dangled from side to side on the parallel bars. Grunting with effort, I did everything demanded of me. I did it with an unabashed eagerness to please those who had power over my life. I wanted to put myself at risk. I wanted to do whatever was supposed to be "good" for me. I believed as absolutely as I have ever believed in anything that rehabilitation would finally placate the hunger of the virus.

But when the therapist commanded me to fall, I cringed. For the prospect of falling terrified me. Every afternoon, as I worked through my prescribed activities, I prayed that I would be able to fall when the session ended. Falling was the most essential "good" of all the "goods" held out for my consideration by my therapist. I believed that. I believed it so intensely that the belief itself was painful. Everything else asked of me was given—and given gladly. I mounted the bus stairs, pushed across the parallel bars until my arms ached with the effort, allowed the medicine ball to pummel me, flailed away at the empty air with my fists because my therapist wanted me to rid myself of the tension within. The slightest sign of approval from those in authority was enough to make me puff with pleasure. Other boys in the ward might not have taken rehabilitation seriously, but I was an eager servant cringing before the promise of approval.

Only, I couldn't fall. As each session ended, I would be led to the mats that took up a full third of the huge room. "It's time," the therapist would say. Dutifully, I would follow her, step after step. Just as dutifully, I would stand on the edge of those two-inch-thick mats, staring down at them until I could feel my body quiver. "All you have to do is let go," my therapist assured me. "The other boys do it. Just let go and fall."

But the prospect of letting go was precisely what terrified me. That the other boys in the ward had no trouble falling added to my shame and terror. I didn't need my therapist to tell me the two-inch-thick mats would keep me from hurting myself. I knew there was virtually no chance of injury when I fell, but that knowledge simply made me more ashamed of a cowardice that was as monumental as it was unexplainable. Had it been able to rid me of my sense of my own cowardice, I would happily have settled for bodily harm. But I was being asked to surrender myself to the emptiness of space, to let go and crash down to the mats below, to feel myself suspended in air when nothing stood between me and the vacuum of the world. *That* was the prospect that overwhelmed me. *That* was what left me sweating with rage and humiliation. The contempt I felt was for my own weakness.

I tried to justify what I sensed could never be justified. Why should I be expected to throw myself into emptiness? Was this sullen terror the price of compensation, the badge of normality? Maybe my refusal to fall embodied some deeper thrust than I could then understand. Maybe I had unconsciously seized upon some fundamental resistance to the forces that threatened to overwhelm me. What did it matter that the ground was covered by the thick mats? The tremors I feared were in my heart and soul.

Shame plagued me—and shame is the older brother to disease. Flushing with shame, I would stare down at the mats. I could feel myself wanting to cry out. But I shriveled at the thought of calling more attention to my cowardice. I would finally hear myself whimper, "I'm sorry. But I can't. I can't let go."

Formless emptiness. A rush of air through which I would plummet toward obliteration. As my "normal" past grew more and more distant, I reached for it more and more desperately, recalling it like some movie whose plot has long since been forgotten but whose scenes continue to comfort through images disconnected from anything but themselves. I remembered that there had been a time when the prospect of falling evoked not terror but joy: football games on the rain-softened autumn turf of Mosholu Parkway, belly-flopping on an American Flyer down its snow-covered slopes in winter, rolling with a pack of friends down one of the steep hills in Bronx Park. Free falls from the past, testifying not to a loss of the self but to an absence of barriers.

My therapist pleaded, ridiculed, cajoled, threatened, bullied. I was sighed over and railed at. But I couldn't let go and fall. I couldn't sell my terror off so cheaply. Ashamed as I was, I wouldn't allow myself to be bullied out of terror.

A month passed—a month of struggle between me and my therapist. Daily excursions to the rehab room, daily practice runs through the future that was awaiting me. The daily humiliation of discovering that one's own fear had been transformed into a public issue, a subject of discussion among the other boys in the ward, seemed unending.

And then, terror simply evaporated. It was as if I had served enough time in that prison. I was ready to move on. One Tuesday afternoon, as my session ended, the therapist walked resignedly alongside me toward the mats. "All right, Leonard. It's time again. All you have to do is let go and fall." Again, I stood above the mats. Only this time, it was as if something beyond my control or understanding had decided to let my body's fall from grace take me down for good. I was not seized by the usual paroxysm of fear. I didn't feel myself break out in a terrified sweat. It was over.

I don't mean that I suddenly felt myself spring into courage. That wasn't what happened at all. The truth was I had simply been worn down into letting go, like a boxer in whose eyes one recognizes

not the flicker of defeat—that issue never having been in doubt—
but the acceptance of defeat. Letting go no longer held my imagination captive. I found myself quite suddenly faced with a necessary
fall—a fall into life.

So it was that I stood above the mat and heard myself sigh and then
felt myself let go, dropping through the quiet air, crutches slipping
off to the sides. What I didn't feel this time was the threat of my
body slipping into emptiness, so mummified by the terror before it
that the touch of air preempted even death. I dropped. I did not
crash. I dropped. I did not collapse. I dropped. I did not plummet. I
felt myself enveloped by a curiously gentle moment in my life. In
that sliver of time before I hit the mat, I was kissed by space.

My body absorbed the slight shock and I rolled onto my back,
braced legs swinging like unguided missiles into the free air, crutches
dropping away to the sides. Even as I fell through the air, I could
sense the shame and fear drain from my soul, and I knew that my
sense of my own cowardice would soon follow. In falling, I had
given myself a new start, a new life.

"That's it!" my therapist triumphantly shouted. "You let go!
And there it is!"

You let go! And there it is! Yes, and you discover not terror but the
only self you are going to be allowed to claim anyhow. You fall free,
and then you learn that those padded mats hold not courage but the
unclaimed self. And if it turned out to be not the most difficult of
tasks, did that make my sense of jubilation any less?

From that moment, I gloried in my ability to fall. Falling became an end in itself. I lost sight of what my therapist had desperately been trying to demonstrate for me—that there was a purpose
in learning how to fall. For she wanted to teach me through the fall
what I would have to face in the future. She wanted to give me a
wholeness I could not give myself. For she knew that mine would be

a future so different from what confronts the "normal" that I had to learn to fall into life in order not to be overwhelmed.

From that day, she urged me to practice falling as if I were a religious disciple being urged by a master to practice spiritual discipline. Letting go meant allowing my body to float into space, to turn at the direction of the fall and follow the urgings of emptiness. For her, learning to fall was learning the most essential of American lessons: how to turn incapacity into capacity.

"You were afraid of hurting yourself," she explained to me. "But that's the beauty of it. When you let go, you can't hurt yourself."

An echo of the streets and playgrounds I called home until I met the virus. American slogans: go with the flow, roll with the punch, slide with the threat until it is no longer a threat. They were simply slogans, and they were all intended to create strength from weakness, a veritable world's fair of compensation.

I returned to the city a year later. By that time, I was a willing convert, one who now secretly enjoyed demonstrating his ability to fall. I enjoyed the surprise that would greet me as I got to my feet, unscathed and undamaged. However perverse it may seem, I felt a certain pleasure when, as I walked with a friend, I felt a crutch slip out of my grasp. Watching the thrust of concern darken his features, I felt myself in control of my own capacity. For falling had become the way my body sought out its proper home. It was an earthbound body, and mine would be an earthbound life. My quest would be for the solid ground beneath me. Falling with confidence, I fell away from terror and fear.

Of course, some falls took me unawares, and I found myself letting go too late or too early. Bruised in ego and sometimes in body, I would pull myself to my feet to consider what had gone wrong. Yet I was essentially untroubled. Such defeats were part of the game, even when they confined me to bed for a day or two afterward. I was an accountant of pain, and sometimes heavier payment was demanded. In my mid-thirties, I walked my two-year-old son's baby-sitter home, tripped on the curbstone, and broke my wrist. At forty-eight, an awkward fall triggered by a carelessly unlocked brace sent me smashing against the bathtub and into surgery for a broken femur. It took four months for me to learn to walk on the crutches all over again. But I learned. I already knew how to fall.

I knew such accidents could be handled. After all, pain was not synonymous with mortality. In fact, pain was insurance against an excessive consciousness of mortality. Pain might validate the specific moment in time, but it didn't have very much to do with the future. I did not yet believe that falling into life had anything to do with falling into death. It was simply a way for me to exercise control over my own existence.

It seems to me today that when I first let my body fall to those mats, I was somehow giving myself the endurance I would need to survive in this world. In a curious way, falling became a way of celebrating what I had lost. My legs were lifeless, useless, but their loss had created a dancing image in whose shadowy gyrations I recognized a strange but potentially interesting new self. I would survive. I knew that now. I could let go, I could fall, and, best of all, I could get up.

To create an independent self, a man had to rid himself of both the myths that nurtured him and the myths that held him back. Learning to fall had been the first lesson in how I yet might live successfully as a cripple. Even disease had its inviolate principles. I understood that the most dangerous threat to the sense of self I needed was an inflated belief in my own capacity. Falling rid a man of excess baggage; it taught him how each of us is dependent on balance.

But what really gave falling legitimacy was the knowledge that I could get to my feet again. That was what taught me the rules of survival. As long as I could pick myself up and stand on my own two feet, brace-bound and crutch-propped as I was, the fall testified to my ability to live in the here and now, to stake my claim as an American who had turned incapacity into capacity. For such a man, falling might well be considered the language of everyday achievement.

. . .

But the day came, as I knew it must, when I could no longer pick myself up. It was then that my passion for symmetry in endings began. On that day, spurred on by another fall, I found myself spinning into the inevitable future.

The day was actually a rainy night in November of 1983. I had just finished teaching at the City College Center for Worker Education, an off-campus degree program for working adults, and had joined some friends for dinner. All of us, I remember, were in a jovial, celebratory mood, although I no longer remember what it was we were celebrating. Perhaps it was simply the satisfaction of being good friends and colleagues at dinner together.

We ate in a Spanish restaurant on Fourteenth Street in Manhattan. It was a dinner that took on, for me at least, the intensity of a time that would assume greater and greater significance as I grew older, one of those watershed moments writers are so fond of. In the dark, rain-swept New York night, change and possibility seemed to drift like a thick fog all around us.

Our mood was still convivial when we left the restaurant around eleven. The rain had slackened off to a soft drizzle and the street glistened beneath the play of light on the wet black creosote. At night, rain in the city has a way of transforming proportion into optimism. The five of us stood around on the slicked-down sidewalk, none of us willing to be the first to break the richness of the mood by leaving.

Suddenly, the crutch in my left hand began to slip out from under me, slowly, almost deliberately, as if the crutch had a mind of its own and had not yet made the commitment that would send me down. Apparently, I had hit a slick patch of city sidewalk, some nub of concrete worn smooth as medieval stone by thousands of shoppers and panhandlers and tourists and students who daily pounded the bargain hustlings of Fourteenth Street.

Instinctively, I at first tried to fight the fall, to seek for balance by pushing off from the crutch in my right hand. But as I recognized that the fall was inevitable, I simply went slack—and for the thousandth time my body sought vindication in its ability to let go and drop. These good friends had seen me fall before. They knew my childish vanities, understood that I still thought of falling as a way to demonstrate my control of the traps and uncertainties that lay in wait for us all.

Thirty-eight years earlier, I had discovered that I could fall into life simply by letting go. Now I made a different discovery—that I could no longer get to my feet by myself. I hit the wet ground and quickly turned over and pushed up, trying to use one of the crutches as a prop to boost myself to my feet, as I had been taught to do as a boy of twelve.

But try as hard as I could, I couldn't get to my feet. It wasn't that I lacked physical strength. I knew that my arms were as powerful as ever as I pushed down on the wet concrete. It had nothing to do with the fact that the street was wet, as my friends insisted later. No, it had to do with a subtle, if mysterious, change in my own sense of rhythm and balance. My body had decided—*and decided on its own, autonomously*—that the moment had come for me to face the question of endings. It was the body that chose its time of recognition.

It was, it seems to me now, a distinctly American moment. It left me pondering limitations and endings and summations. It left me with the curiously buoyant sense that mortality had quite suddenly made itself a felt presence rather than the rhetorical strategy used by the poets and novelists I taught to my students. This was what writers had in mind when they spoke of the truly common fate, this sense of ending coming to one unbidden. This had brought with it my impassioned quest for symmetry. As I lay on the wet ground— no more than a minute or two—all I could think of was how much I wanted my life to balance out. It was as if I were staring into a future in which time itself had evaporated.

Here was a clear, simple perception, and there was nothing mystical about it. There are limitations we recognize and those that recognize us. My friends, who had nervously been standing around while I tried to get to my feet, finally asked if they could help me up. "You'll have to," I said. "I can't get up any other way."

Two of them pulled me to my feet while another jammed the crutches beneath my arms, as the therapist and the two bracemakers had done almost four decades earlier. When I was standing, they proceeded to joke about my sudden incapacity in that age-old way men of all ages have, as if words might codify loss and change and time's betrayal. I joined in the joking. But what I really wanted was to go home and contemplate this latest fall in the privacy of my apartment. The implications were clear: I would never again be an eater of salt, I would also never again get to my feet on my own. A part of my life had ended. But that didn't depress me. In fact, I felt almost as exhilarated as I had thirty-eight years earlier when my body surrendered to the need to let go and I fell into life.

Almost four years have passed since I fell on the wet sidewalk of Fourteenth Street. I suppose it wasn't a particularly memorable fall. It wasn't even particularly significant to anyone who had not once fallen into life. But it was inevitable, the first time I had let go into a time when it would no longer even be necessary to let go.

It was a fall that left me with the knowledge that I could no longer pick myself up. That meant I now needed the help of others as I had not needed their help before. It was a fall that left me burning with this strange passion for symmetry, this desire to balance my existence. When the day comes, I want to be able to fall into my death as nakedly as I once had to fall into my life.

Do not misunderstand me. I am not seeking a way out of mortality, for I believe in nothing more strongly than I believe in the permanency of endings. I am not looking for a way out of this life, a life I continue to find immensely enjoyable—even if I can no longer pull myself to my own two feet. Of course, a good deal in my life has changed. For one thing, I am increasingly impatient with those who claim to have no use for endings of any sort. I am also increasingly embarrassed by the thought of the harshly critical adolescent I was, self-righteously convinced that the only way for a man to go to his end was by kicking and screaming.

But these are, I suppose, the kinds of changes any man or woman of forty or fifty would feel. Middle-aged skepticism is as natural as adolescent acne. In my clearer, less passionate moments, I can even laugh at my need for symmetry in beginnings and endings as well as my desire to see my own eventual death as a line running parallel to my life. Even in mathematics, let alone life, symmetry is sometimes too neat, too closed off from the way things actually work. After all, it took me a full month before I could bring myself to let go and fall into life.

I no longer talk about how one can seize a doctrine of compensation from disease. I don't talk about it, but it still haunts me. In my heart, I believe it offers a man the only philosophy by which he can actually live. It is the only philosophy that strips away both spiritual mumbo jumbo and the procrustean weight of existential anxiety. In the final analysis, a man really is what a man does.

Believing as I do, I wonder why I so often find myself trying to frame a perspective that will prove adequate to a proper sense of ending. Perhaps that is why I find myself sitting in a bar with a friend, trying to explain to him all that I have learned from falling. "There must be a time," I hear myself tell him, "when a man has the right to stop thinking about falling."

"Sure," my friend laughs. "Four seconds before he dies."

daniel d. baxter, m.d.

In this opening chapter of his book, the author helps
the reader experience the Spellman Center AIDS memorial service on two levels—from the distance of an
observer in the congregation and, more intimately,
through fleeting memories of his former patients. He is
particularly effective while listing sentence fragments
of lost patients and recalling moments or details about
each of them.

in memoriam

Locus iste a Deo factus est, inaestimabile sacramentum, irreprehensibilis est. This dwelling is God's handiwork: a mystery beyond all price that cannot be spoken against.

—TEXT FROM THE MASS FOR THE DEDICATION OF A CHURCH

Every three months, with the change of seasons, a remarkable memorial service is held in the small chapel of St. Clare's Hospital in New York City. Organized by the hospital's Spellman Center for HIV-Related Diseases, this quiet service is intended, in the words of Sister Pascal Conforti, "to remember and celebrate the lives of our friends who have died and left us." The "friends" Sister Pascal speaks of were patients who have died from AIDS.

Centrally located on the ground floor of this aging hospital, the gemlike chapel of St. Clare's is neither opulent nor austere in decor. The founding Franciscan sisters designed it earlier this century as a place for both celebration and meditation, not religious ostentation. Inside the entrance doorway, competing for precious space, are a closet-sized confessional, a small basin of holy water, and a miniature Wurlitzer organ. Three tiny stained-glass windows filter amber light onto narrow wooden pews and reddish marble walls, which are crammed with small plaques denoting the fourteen stations of the cross. Framing a dramatic backdrop to the slightly elevated altar is a life-size oil painting of the glorification of St. Clare, St. Francis, and Our Lady of Mount Carmel. Despite the chapel's compactness—its total floor space might accommodate a regulation-size tennis court—an ethereal airiness suffuses throughout, perhaps because of the vaulted blue ceiling, or because of the countless memories contained within its walls. Glowing warmly in late afternoon sunlight, the chapel of St. Clare's is an inviting little space—a tranquil sanctuary from the drab and fearsome AIDS wards that surround it on all sides.

Participating in this quarterly memorial service is a cross section of the Spellman Center staff: social workers, nurses, physician assistants, volunteers, secretaries, administrators. Although family and friends of the deceased are always invited, few are ever able to come, and most of the dozen or so people in attendance are Spellman employees. There are often more people at a Greenwich Village memorial service for one gay man than there are at St. Clare's thirty minutes of remembrance for the scores of its AIDS patients. As a Spellman physician, I go to these memorial services with both anticipation and trepidation: while exceedingly important to commemorate, the memories of former patients are sometimes too intense to revisit after an already difficult day on my inpatient AIDS ward. But I am always drawn to the Spellman memorial service because I feel it reminds me why I must be an AIDS doctor.

Starting at four with a quiet musical prelude on the chapel's organ, the service varies little from season to season. Sister Pascal gives a brief introductory welcome, followed by a staff member's reading of a meditative poem or short spiritual story. Then, to musical accompaniment, a procession of three or four staff marches to the altar, where they open the Book of Remembrance and light the memorial candle. Thereupon commences the heart of the service, the Reading of Names: quietly—*reverently*—the staff members alternate in reading aloud from the Book of Remembrance the names of the fifty or so patients who have died on the Spellman AIDS service over the prior three months. There are many names like Jose, Yolanda, Juan, Maria, and Hector—not the names of middle-class gay white males or of people listed in the *Times* obituary columns. These are society's poor and marginalized: the prisoners and ex-prisoners, the drug users and ex-drug users, the prostitutes, the homeless, the unwanted, or the forgotten . . . unwanted or forgotten, that is, until they came to St. Clare's and its Spellman Center.

With the slow reading of the names of the dead, memories wash over the audience, engulfing everyone in a spectrum of emotions. Each name evokes numerous, extraordinary remembrances and impressions: the patient's personality and idiosyncrasies, or aspects of the patient's disease and course of illness, or his or her emotional response to dying from AIDS. No sooner does one name spark a cascade of memories than another name is called and the process repeats. One name may recall the image of an ever-attentive mother—or sister or lover or spouse or friend—holding bedside vigil for his or her loved one. Another name might bring forth the haunting picture of an emaciated prisoner dying alone, far from his family in Puerto Rico. Yet another might evoke that patient's engaging smile and sense of humor, as she would playfully joke with her doctors and nurses. As the Reading of Names solemnly proceeds, the mind recalls random, even trivial images—a family photo on a patient's bedside stand, a patient's favorite dress or colorful turn of phrase, a handmade quilt that always covered a patient's bed, a small picture of the Blessed Virgin a worried mother taped on the wall of her only son's room, or one of a thousand other minor details of a patient's life on the Spellman service.

Some of the names are of patients who died on Unit 3A, my own AIDS ward; others are of people who passed away on adjacent Spellman floors. Even so, these latter patients are largely well known to me, since I may have cared for them on an earlier admission or heard their cases discussed at Spellman's TB rounds or morning report. Indeed, as Sister Pascal says, most Spellman patients have become friends to the staff.

"Hector R." . . . the crunching sound of ribs cracking during a cardiac resuscitation so violent that his teddy bear is inadvertently pushed off the bed onto the floor, into a pool of mal—

"Joey S." . . . taped on the walls around his bed are the many handmade get-well cards and drawings from his little nephews and nieces, whose hope for their Uncle Joey's recovery contrasts so graphically with the bloody sce—

"Ricardo C." . . . his worried mother's refusals to understand her only son's terminal condition, as she would endlessly pace about his hospital room all hours of the day and night, nervously reacting to his every moan, his every—

"Rosa M." . . .

And so it goes: during each memorial service, my mind is brusquely whipsawed from one universe of memories to another, as the somber, rhythmic recitation of names proceeds with three-second regularity.

After the last name is read from the Book of Remembrance, an almost palpable emotional exhaustion ripples through the chapel. We sense that the awesome memories we just felt could only be encompassed by an infinite intelligence and love, far beyond mortal grasp. As the four staff close the Book of Remembrance and file back into the audience, I am relieved that the emotional roller coaster has ended, but am uneasy over the truncated memories that I feel I *must* yet ponder and take to heart.

After the Reading of Names, someone else reads another poem or brief Bible passage, and then two or three staff members or relatives come forward and recount "Stories of Remembering"—anecdotes or impressions about patients who have most affected them. A Spellman volunteer relates how her acceptance and understanding of death were enhanced by a dying patient's courage. A social worker speaks of a previously fragmented family reunited by a dying patient's love. A physician assistant, an avid Yankees fan, tells how he single-handedly took another fan—his patient with terminal, AIDS-related lymphoma—from his hospital bed to a Yankees game a week before he died. A family member, barely holding back tears, relives happier times, when a loved one was active and well. Without exception, Spellman patients are remembered as vibrant individuals—never as diseased people dying from AIDS in hospital beds, but rather as *people who have much to teach about life and living.*

Finally, the program closes with a song or hymn, followed by a brief prayer by the hospital priest, Father Jack. The entire service lasts no more than thirty minutes or so. It is unrehearsed and unfinished; at times awkward gaffes occur. Sometimes the background music warbles off-key—the Wurlitzer is *very* old—or the 1950s public address system sputters on and off. Occasionally, a speaker's meditative story will ramble on, never quite coming to the point. During Stories of Remembering, tears frequently cut short a friend's reminiscences. Yet as simpleminded as it might seem to a cynical outsider, an unspeakable sadness and intensity permeates every Spellman memorial service.

Immediately after every service, a punch-and-cookies reception is held in the hospital's ancient cafeteria, where relatives and friends in attendance can visit with the staff who cared for their loved ones. The reunion can be bittersweet: most of the friends and family have not been back to St. Clare's, or spoken with their loved one's caregivers, since his or her death. There are often more tears at the reception than in the chapel, as memories of the deceased are relived. But always standing close by, ready with a supportive word—or a hug, if necessary—is Sister Pascal, the director of pastoral care and Spellman's guardian angel. Pascal radiates transcendent strength and serenity, renewing the flagging spirits of family and staff alike. As I watch her move among everyone at the reception, I marvel at her all-inclusive compassion. It is like seeing Schweitzer quietly working in his Central African hospital, or Jane Addams in Hull House. Pascal likes to boast that for all its many problems, St. Clare's Spellman Center has "soul," due in no small part to her devotion to its patients and its healing mission—"a mystery beyond all price that cannot be spoken against."

After twenty minutes or so, the reception breaks up, and the family and friends return home to continue with their lives, which sadly often entail looking after yet another friend or relative who has AIDS and may someday have his or her name called out from the Book of Remembrance. The staff drift back to their floors to finish up the day's work.

I leave each memorial service with a feeling of incompleteness—an ill-defined sadness, an uneasy longing. There is *never* enough time to pause and relive each deceased patient's story, to apply each patient's experiences with AIDS to my own life. Walking home, I feel compelled to revisit many of the names recited earlier. Hours later, the Reading of Names still reverberates in my head as I reflect upon the protean lessons about life each name of the dead speaks to me.

rebecca mcclanahan

"Liferower" is a parallel narrative in which, on a very basic level, the reader shares a physical experience—an intense session on a liferower. Simultaneously, in fits and starts and with twists and turns (the proportions of a fetus, her pregnant sister, etc.), a nagging intimacy is revealed. The revelation is effectively authentic—exactly the scattered way in which unshakable memories return to us (haphazardly . . . but nonetheless powerfully) in life.

liferower

There I am on the Liferower screen, the computerized woman in the tiny boat; and the little woman rowing below me is my pacer. We look exactly alike, except she does not get tired. Her strokes are even and unchanging. I aim for thirty-three pulls per minute, but if I rest even a second between strokes, I fall behind. I want to train my heart, to make it stronger.

"Keep up with the pacer," blinks the sign on the screen. "Use your legs. Keep your back straight."

You row with your whole body, not just your arms. There is a leaning into, then a pulling away. The filling and the emptying. Systole, diastole. The iambic lub and dub—and sometimes a murmur, a leak in the heart. My father's valve has been replaced with plastic that clicks when he overexerts himself. Bad hearts run in our family. An infant sister died of a congenital ailment; another sister nearly died from a myocardial infection contracted while she was giving birth to her second child. I have no children. Which is why I am free to come here to the Y and row my heart out three times a week. Aside from a husband who can take care of himself—as most second husbands are able to do—I have no one to worry about. This thought disturbs me, wakes me at night. If I have no one to care for, who will care for me? When I was small I shared a bedroom with an old woman, my mother's childless aunt, who had nowhere else to go. I have fourteen nephews and nieces. Will any of them claim me? Each month from my paycheck I put away more than I can afford, insurance against what time will bring. According to surveys, women

fear old age more than men do—the poverty, the loneliness. And the hearts of women beat faster and harder, both waking and sleeping, than the hearts of men.

"Keep up the good work. You are one boat ahead."

From the shoreline a crowd of miniature fans wave me on to victory. Each time I pull the rowing rope, the little woman on the screen moves her cartoon arms. The oar dips and lifts and a ripple of water sloshes across the screen, accompanied by a *whoosh* that's intended to sound like rushing water, but sounds more like the breath of a woman in labor: in through the nose, out through the mouth. *Whoosh, whoosh.* In the delivery room I smoothed my sister's clenched fist and watched the electrocardiograph as twin waves danced across the screen—the rise and fall of mother and daughter. The heart is a double pump composed of four separate rooms. If I divide my age into four equal chambers, I am eleven again. It is the year I begin to bleed, the year my mother pushes my sister into the world.

I pump my legs and pull the rope. In a large open area beside the rowing machines, a yoga class begins. The instructor greets the sun, breathing in *prana,* the invisible life force: in through the nose, out through the mouth. The other women follow, open their mouths on the first half of the healing mantra *Om.* I like the sound of *forty-four*—the "O" bell tone, sonorous and deep. The echo. I don't like the way it looks—two fours standing shoulder to shoulder, square and bony, each built from single sticks of *one* that could easily collapse. Like an awkward stork perched precariously in midair, tipping on one thin leg. The yoga master has now become a tree—arms branching into finger leaves high above her head, one leg balanced against a thigh, the other the root sinking her deep into imaginary soil. *You can't learn balance,* she is saying. *You can only allow it.* The heart is controlled by two opposing bundles of nerves, the sympathetic and the parasympathetic. One slows the beat, the other quickens it. Thus, balance is achieved through a back-and-forth dance, two mutually antagonistic forces pushing simultaneously against and for one another.

On the screen, red buoys bob between me and my pacer, marking off the miles in tenths: one point six, one point seven. The water rolls beneath us and in the distance a miniature skyline looms. It's the kind of city a child might construct from Lego pieces, chunks of towers and boxy buildings in the shape of bar graphs a math teacher draws on the blackboard. What goes up must come down. My Y locker combination—32-22-32—is easy to remember because those were my measurements half a lifetime ago, when I was being fitted for my first wedding dress. The dress, which my mother saved, hangs in her guest room closet. The marriage lasted three years, three years longer than it should have because I was determined not to fail. My mother was my measure, my pacer, and when my husband began turning from me, I rowed faster and faster toward him. I would work harder, cook more of his favorite foods, steam his khakis with a cleaner pleat.

"Lean into the stroke. Keep up with the pacer. You are three boats behind."

On the rower beside mine, a young woman pumps with long tanned legs and pulls with lean muscled arms that she probably believes will never soften. Her body is something she counts on—the belly flat, the skin snug and elastic as the spandex leotard glowing in oranges and greens, the neon parrot hues of one whose life does not yet depend on camouflage. The weight instructor, a short, well-built man about my age, bends to speak to her, to comment on her form and technique. He does not see me. When he leaves, she watches her reflection in the floor-to-ceiling mirror as if her body belongs to someone else. Her forehead is prematurely lined with worry; she is not enjoying this. Nearby, the yoga master assumes the lion pose, crouched and ready. She bares her teeth, lifts her mane into the air.

"Use your legs. Keep your back straight. You are five boats behind."

The heart is a hollow muscle housed in a slippery, loose-fitting sac and protected by three layers of membranes. Its size varies from person to person, but is approximately the size of a clenched fist. At five weeks a fetus is barely eight millimeters long, but already its heart is beating on its own. When my sister had her first sonogram, I watched on the screen the undulating blur that would become my niece. The heart cells were already in place, all the cells my niece would need for the rest of her life. Her heartbeat sounded like a train roaring through a tunnel. A child comes into this world hammering its heart out, 160 beats per minute, a teletype machine tapping its urgent message. And deep in the aortic chamber of each adult there survives a hole, the foramen ovale, remnant of the place where blood passed through the fetal heart.

The child I chose against would have been born into the cramped space of my life between marriages. I still ask myself how it could have happened. *Things happen.* You wake one morning and you know. Your tender breasts tell you and the flush across your cheeks and the feeling of something larger and smaller than yourself moving inside you. Time passes, liquid as a dream, and one morning, because you are alone and your life is a rented room, you make the call. And the next day when it's over and the nurse takes the gauze from between your teeth, the doctor, who is kind and slightly plump, his forehead lined from having seen too much, holds up a glass bottle filled with something bright and red. "This is pregnancy," he says, believing it's for your own good. "Don't let this happen again." And then it's over, it's done. But your legs are still trembling and your tongue is bleeding from where you bit down and missed.

Five boats ahead of me, the pacer slides over the finish line, leaving red buoys bobbing in her wake. I place my fingertips on my carotid artery and begin the count that will bring me back to myself. Easing up on the rope, I pump slower, slower, my boat cruising past the crowd of bystanders waving from the shoreline. The yoga master begins her descent into this world, shifting from eagle to fish to cat to flower, shape by shape removing herself, moving toward a place that knows no shape. When she reaches it, she bows to the altar of Sadguru, the larger self that dwells within the smallest place. Forehead pressed to the ground, she assumes the child position:

shoulders down, knees folded to belly, hands and feet at rest, ears open to the slightest sound. The music of a single heartbeat is actually two-part harmony, a duet sung by opposing valves, the low-pitched *lub* of the atrioventricular and the higher pitched *dub* as the semilunar closes down. The yoga master opens her mouth on "O" and the others follow, float on this communal pond until together their lips close on the hum, and one by one, their single breaths give out.

anatole broyard

As unlikely as it may seem to be intoxicated by the
specter of your own death, Broyard is quite convincing
because he focuses on a narrow line of elation. He
doesn't alibi or make excuses for his obvious illogic; he
admits to the weakness of his convictions and qualifies
his elation by explaining his feelings at that particular
moment in time.

intoxicated by my illness

So much of a writer's life consists of assumed suffering, rhetorical suffering, that I felt something like relief, even elation, when the doctor told me that I had cancer of the prostate. Suddenly there was in the air a rich sense of crisis, real crisis, yet one that also contained echoes of ideas like the crisis of language, the crisis of literature, or of personality. It seemed to me that my existence, whatever I thought, felt, or did, had taken on a kind of meter, as in poetry, or in taxis.

When you learn that your life is threatened, you can turn toward this knowledge or away from it. I turned toward it. It was not a choice but an automatic shifting of gears, a tacit agreement between my body and my brain. I thought that time had tapped me on the shoulder, that I had been given a real deadline at last. It wasn't that I believed the cancer was going to kill me, even though it had spread beyond the prostate—it could probably be controlled, either by radiation or hormonal manipulation. No, what struck me was the startled awareness that one day something, whatever it might be, was going to interrupt my leisurely progress. It sounds trite, yet I can only say that I realized for the first time that I don't have forever.

Time was no longer innocuous, nothing was casual anymore. I understood that living itself had a deadline. Like the book I had been working on—how sheepish I would feel if I couldn't finish it. I had promised it to myself and to my friends. Though I wouldn't say this out loud, I had promised it to the world. All writers privately think this way.

When my friends heard I had cancer, they found me surprisingly cheerful and talked about my courage. But it has nothing to do with courage, at least not for me. As far as I can tell, it's a question of desire. I'm filled with desire—to live, to write, to do everything. Desire itself is a kind of immortality. While I've always had trouble concentrating, I now feel as concentrated as a diamond, or a microchip.

I remember a time in the 1950s when I tried to talk a friend of mine named Jules out of committing suicide. He had already made one attempt and when I went to see him he said, "Give me a good reason to go on living." He was thirty years old.

I saw what I had to do. I started to sell life to him, like a real estate agent. Just look at the world, I said. How can you not be curious about it? The streets, the houses, the trees, the shops, the people, the movement, and the stillness. Look at the women, so appealing, each in her own way. Think of all the things you can do with them, the places you can go together. Think of books, paintings, music. Think of your friends.

While I was talking I wondered, Am I telling Jules the truth? He didn't think so, because he put his head in the oven a week later. As for me, I don't know whether I believed what I said or not, because I just went on behaving like everybody else. But I believe it now. When my wife made me a hamburger the other day I thought it was the most fabulous hamburger in the history of the world.

With this illness one of my recurrent dreams has finally come true. Several times in the past I've dreamed that I had committed a crime—or perhaps I was only accused of a crime, it's not clear. When brought to trial I refused to have a lawyer—I got up instead and made an impassioned speech in my own defense. This speech was so moving that I could feel myself tingling with it. It was inconceivable that the jury would not acquit me—only each time, I woke before the verdict. Now cancer is the crime I may or may not have committed, and the eloquence of being alive, the fervor of the survivor, is my best defense.

The way my friends have rallied around me is wonderful. They remind me of a flock of birds rising from a body of water into the sunset. If that image seems a bit extravagant, or tinged with satire, it's because I can't help thinking there's something comical about my friends' behavior, all these witty men suddenly saying pious, inspirational things.

They are not intoxicated as I am by my illness, but sobered. Since I refused to, they've taken on the responsibility of being serious. They appear abashed, or chagrined, in their sobriety. Stripped of their playfulness these pals of mine seem plainer, homelier—even older. It's as if they had all gone bald overnight.

Yet one of the effects of their fussing over me is that I feel vivid, multicolored, sharply drawn. On the other hand—and this is ungrateful—I remain outside of their solicitude, their love and best wishes. I'm isolated from them by the grandiose conviction that I am the healthy person and they are the sick ones. Like an existential hero, I have been cured by the truth while they still suffer the nausea of the uninitiated.

I've had eight-inch needles thrust into my belly where I could feel them tickling my metaphysics. I've worn Pampers. I've been licked by the flames and my sense of self has been singed. Sartre was right: you have to live each moment as if you're prepared to die.

Now at last I understand the conditional nature of the human condition. Yet, unlike Kierkegaard and Sartre, I'm not interested in the irony of my position. Cancer cures you of irony. Perhaps my irony was all in my prostate. A dangerous illness fills you with adrenaline and makes you feel very smart. I can afford now, I said to myself, to draw conclusions. All those grand generalizations toward which I have been building for so many years are finally taking shape. As I look back at how I used to be, it seems to me that an intellectual is a person who thinks that the classical clichés don't apply to him, that he is immune to homely truths. I know better now. I see everything with a summarizing eye. Nature is a terrific editor.

In the first stages of my illness I couldn't sleep, urinate, or defecate—the word "ordeal" comes to mind. Then when my doctor changed all this and everything worked again, what a voluptuous pleasure it was. With a cry of joy I realized how marvelous it is simply to function. My body, which in the last decade or two had become a familiar, no longer thrilling old flame, was reborn as a brand-new infatuation.

I realize of course that this elation I feel is just a phase, just a rush of consciousness, a splash of perspective, a hot flash of ontological alertness. But I'll take it, I'll use it. I'll use everything I can while I wait for the next phase. Illness is primarily a drama and it should be possible to enjoy it as well as to suffer it. I see now why the romantics were so fond of illness—the sick man sees everything as metaphor. In this phase I'm infatuated with my cancer. It stinks of revelation.

As I look ahead, I feel like a man who has awakened from a long afternoon nap to find the evening stretched out before him. I'm reminded of D'Annunzio, the Italian poet, who said to a duchess he had just met at a party in Paris, "Come, we will have a profound evening." Why not? I see the balance of my life—everything comes in images now—as a beautiful paisley shawl thrown over a grand piano.

Why a paisley shawl, precisely? Why a grand piano? I have no idea. That's the way the situation presents itself to me. I have to take my imagery along with my medicine.

susan l. adkins

The structural elements of "The Strength of Bald-Headed Women" are easy to appreciate: (1) Using the lady wrestler as a way to compel and drive the reader, (2) anchoring the scene and echoing selective family details as a subtle but effective record of two separate time frames. The magic (healing) moment occurs when the sister reveals the father by doffing her wig.

the strength of
bald-headed women

Holy ritual ruled on Saturday nights just as strongly as it did on Sunday mornings. With sunset came the traditional procession to the front porch where my parents, my sister, and I fit ourselves into stiff-backed wooden rocking chairs. As the female head of household, Granny served sweaty glasses of Royal Crown Cola that were sipped slowly in time with the give and take of the weekly family communion. Despite this syrupy liquid, all those who congregated there blistered their mouths on Granny's salty popcorn while contemplating the great mysteries of life. It was as though concentrated levels of sodium forced truths to the surface.

Granny's wood-frame house sat on cheap land. The front yard climbed straight up the side of the hill where a narrow paved road wound its way toward places called Horsepasture and Blackberry. Not a minute passed without a Chevy or Ford squealing round the curve and by the house. As Granny drank down the last of her cola, she always counted the cars that passed. My sister and I would sigh with boredom as she wondered aloud how God was going to get rid of all those cars when he decided to destroy the world on his second coming. Our mother always suspected Granny silently gave thanks for such dilemmas. Anything that might delay Judgment Day was welcome.

Across town, other porches were busy, too. While the glow from Walter Cronkite's six o'clock report might be heating up a few front rooms, most families were cooling outside, watching the street with eyes honed to the darkness. Fathers snored and grunted occasionally in the porch swings, mothers strained to hear muffled conversations that ricocheted up and down the "hollers" of the town, and children dreamed of their eventual escape from southwest Virginia. No tourists ever took a detour to ride through Fieldale. If they had, everyone would have sensed their presence like a barometer falling before an approaching thunderstorm. So when a road show of professional wrestlers decided to stop over for one Saturday night, the pressure behind our inner ears set off alarms.

On the night of the match, the hills emptied out and the town actually had traffic. My family all refused to go with me to the contest, but Granny still kept tally of the invading cars and also studied one of the hundreds of flyers we had found stapled to almost every light pole across a three-county area. These were black-on-white handbills with just words—no blurred photos outlining the flabby physiques of King William and his opponents, the Titan Twins tag team. No, the flyer was just block-lettered text announcing the match. The small print at the bottom promised that a bald-headed woman would wrestle that night.

From the top row of the bleachers, I first saw her as a white blur moving at the nucleus of a tight circle of featureless men. At the time, it reminded me of a porch spider—a puffy, white, bulging head with too many legs to move very fast. So it surprised me when they rushed her past the gate, through the swarms of wild children, and in between the rows of three-dollar seats that hugged the ringside. They protected her so well that no one got a glimpse of her until she actually stepped into the ring. A black cape cocooned her tall, thick, muscular body from neck to ankle, and a white triangle of cloth covered the broad crown of her head. Much to my surprise, the scarf that only partially hid her baldness was so undersized it could not be tied. Instead it simply lay unattached but firmly in position across the top of her head.

Insects hovered, sucking their energy from the overhead lights, and the crowd of people tore off jackets in the cool night air. They glowed red with a sweat that smelled raw and inflamed. Eyes fixed on the bald head that crowned a plain woman's smooth complexion, arched brows, and thin silent lips. Psyches rebelled. "Look at that ugly thing," screamed a man seated two rows in front of me. Nature took charge and their bodies belched in collective shock as the bald-headed woman and her opponent moved around each other—two primates bent toward aggression.

Their feet and legs were squeezed into thin, skinny appendages by tightly laced black leather boots. Above the lacing their calves and thighs sprouted cartoon style with muscles that flexed and reflexed up and down their crouched legs. Feet braced wide for combat. Arms extended and curled out from their sides, and palms wrapped up into hammer fists ready to pummel and bang pain into vertebra, stomach, and kidneys. The opponent's hair blazed beneath the strong stadium lights and shot flames of peroxide blond. Meanwhile, the bald-headed woman's face locked in a gaze I could not read.

Body slams, back drops, double wrist locks, flying head scissors and tackles, plus hammerlocks and knee lifts followed, but still the scarf stayed in place. Blondie's face twisted while the bald woman's cheek muscles tightened. The crowd booed and threw empty cups and hot dog wrappers at the freak who moved with grace and power while they cheered for the blond wrestler who fell and stumbled and was extraordinarily inept at removing a small scarf that had no visible means of attachment. Only after making a rear approach, Blondie finally snatched the scarf easily from the pate of the bald head. The people howled up into the night sky, wiped the sweat from their faces, and promptly lost interest.

Factory workers and farmers had metamorphosed into a rabid crowd that screamed for the scalp of a woman. Though she fought hard, once exposed, the bald-headed woman had stood straight and stared silently down at us. I was glad Granny had not been part of this. She would not have understood anymore than I did the bald woman and her scarf or the crowd's reaction. No, I wanted to ask my older sister whom I trusted to explain the bizarre, but when I arrived home late, I found her facedown in a feather pillow, asleep with a white cotton sheet pulled up round her neck. Only the back of her head was visible—a mass of black hair swollen and pocked with pink curlers. Perhaps I asked her the next day, but my memory is severed here.

Today we meet at my sister's house. It is large and brick—of French colonial design with a wildflower garden down the back. Three acres of woodland isolate it from the golf course that runs in front and behind. Still, it sits on the side of a hill with a road passing high above. Not a minute goes by without a Honda or Volvo squealing around the curve and by the house. It is May and the sweat of summer only threatens in late afternoon. Nights are still cool and hospitable. It will be weeks yet before the heat and humidity smother us. Dan Rather is on the television, but we click the remote and he becomes quiet and disappears.

My sister spreads mayo flat and even to all four corners of the slice of wheat bread. Layers of turkey come next, crowned with a wiry green leaf and a circle of yellow tomato. Everyone else is either stirring or opening or stacking or tasting or pouring something. I stand by the cold oven, watching the group's choreography and my sister's face. Framed by a blue scarf, her complexion is smooth and accented by arched brows. With thin, almost silent lips, she controls the rhythm, the step, the partnering—a quiet word about the plates, a point to the knife drawer, a yes, a no, a smile, a laugh, a familiar sarcasm.

She rattles down a dozen plates from the cupboard and teases her son aloud. He smiles and then laughs, but his eyes do not follow. Her steady left hand picks at the utensil drawer. When she turns her back, our mother's eyes rise from the celery board like heat-seeking missiles. Small and gray and sharp, they lock onto the back of my sister's neck where a remaining chaff of hair waits to detach and fall. Suddenly my mother's gaze is driven in reverse and back onto the cutting board where she carves the celery into pulp. My sister turns and looks straight at her, "Have I counted right? There are nine of us, right?"

We sit around the rectangular table with eyes burrowing into potato salad. Brother passes the salt to sister who sets it next to brother-in-law. "Someone start the fruit salad," my sister commands, and three pairs of hands and arms reach out for the bright bowl of strawberries and orange and melon. Eyes fixate with relief on the colors and the shapes as the deep dish is traded from one to the other. Talk of last night's rainstorm rides around the table with the glass tray of sweet pickles, and everyone studies their dwindling sandwiches as though they have never seen a tomato before.

Something in my sister's voice unlocks our eyes, and we all look up. "Do you want to take a look at Daddy?" With that she pulls the scarf from her head, showing us her baldness. Only a few strands of gray hang on in irregular patches. Her mouth stretches into a smile, revealing the gold crowns hidden in the back of her mouth. "Don't I look just like him." Eyes and thoughts settle on that bald head. We forget hospitals and doctors and howl with laughter in the afternoon heat, wipe the perspiration from our faces, and promptly agree she has more hair than Daddy did his entire adult life.

After sunset, we join each other on the deck. We fit ourselves into lounge chairs—all white and plastic. Tall glasses of Coke sit secure in cork-lined coasters, and my sister's daughter rips open microwaved bags of popcorn—the greasy, salty kind Granny always loved. Headlights cut through the darkness and our mother stops, "That's the sixth car that's passed in the last ten minutes." My sister sighs. I sigh. As the salt begins to fester along the wrinkled edges of our lips, we all begin to feel a rush of sodium circulating through our veins. The smooth complexion and arched brows of a woman wrestler surface in my memory and with them a belief in the strength of bald-headed women.

katherine russel rich

In this realistic profile of the all-consuming roller coaster triggered by her battle to survive cancer, Katherine Russel Rich endures, among other things, chemotherapy, drugs, bone marrow transplantation— and fear of failure and death. Her triumph is never re- solved in any singular moment; rather it is ongoing and remarkable.

rock

Every day for four months I wear a hairpiece, then one day I don't. You wanted to be the kind of woman who would go out without a wig, I think one Sunday night. Well, here's your chance. The following morning, I'm at my desk bald. In truth, I'm not demonstrating courage or defiance or the fact that cancer patients have nothing to be ashamed of. I'm hot. Spring had exploded like a cheer, and summer has followed with its own Bronx variety. New York is a hermetically sealed cauldron, the sludgy air made leaden by pollution.

By now, July, I'm trudging through mornings in a haze of exhaustion, then going home early and drowning in sleep. I'm fed up with being sick, of being perpetually hounded by inconvenience, like when I go to the gym and have to worry about my hair sliding sideways. Once, in the weight room, where all the pumped-up juice boys were hoisting and grunting, I lay down on a bench with some three-pound weights and my wig promptly fell off, exposing my scrubby head. Mortified, I jammed it back on, but I wasn't sure if it was on straight. Without a mirror, I couldn't tell. "You'd better move it," the guy next to me said. "Okay," I muttered, repositioning the bangs. A silence followed. "Excuse me," he said, "I'm going to lift this"—and he patted weights the size of wagon wheels, hanging on a rack near my ears—"so I think you better move the bench, or it could come down on you." My hairdo, when I sat up, was cocked to the left, as if it were turning toward the wall in embarrassment.

"I thought that was bad hair, not a wig!" Diego exclaimed the first time he saw it, when he came to pick me up after an MRI.

"Diego, censor yourself," I said.

"No, no, it's good," he said. "I did not think that was a wig, only bad hair."

The wig was doing half the job. "I am so sorry I said that," Michelle had begun one morning call. Now that I'm on chemo, many of my phone conversations start this way: *I'm so sorry I said: That thing last night about NutraSweet being carcinogenic. That Tina's mother is sick. That I got a free shampoo sample in the mail.* People's voices quaver as if they've been up half the night kicking themselves in bed. It's only my nicest friends who say these things, which are always inscrutable to me until we've finely deconstructed our last conversation. *Remember, remember, I said* . . . They sound so distressed, I am very careful never to laugh.

Michelle, in this instance, was so sorry that at a baby shower she'd said my hair looked longer. "Your wig is so natural, I forgot."

Really, not a problem, I tell her. But when we hang up, I consider: This ratty toupee does look like I've grown it myself, and it does look pretty bad. Wouldn't I be better off without it? Not long after, I lose the hair. It's as easy as floating into a deeper realm of the sea.

On the street, almost no one gives me a second look. In my world, almost everyone cheers me on. "Sinead!" they say. Or "You're so brave." Or "You really do look beautiful." I love it. It's a shortcut to bolstering, which I really need. Someone from the support group has died, someone my age, and I'm lost in chemo, unable to go back on my decision to stop the hormones and start nuking, not sure I can go forward anymore. My bald head represents my refusal to let cancer oppress me, I try telling myself, but the warrior stuff won't fly anymore, not even with me. Lambrakis has called to say I've cleared the tests, I'm in, I'm going to have a transplant. I'm horribly and profoundly scared.

That's when Laura calls up and offers to teach me to meditate. Someone I know through the magazine, she's had several bouts of breast cancer and is doing fine, a state she attributes, in part, to meditation. If the opinion comes from her, I respect it. Laura's written a book about the brain, knows her Eastern and Western religions, and when she talks about cancer as a spiritual journey, she's smart enough not to sound like she's burping up a bad New Age book. Meditation bores me silly, but I have a whole lot of time on my hands, so I say, "Sure, great." After explaining the techniques, she gives me the rules: Practice twice a day, phone in once a week.

On Wednesday nights I phone, and we fall into great, roiling conversations, like two anchoresses sprung from our cells. We rush past meditation to get to cancer, theology, and death. As badly as I needed to, until she broached it, I hadn't figured out a way to talk about death with anyone, unspeakable as it is in this culture. You can't exactly turn to your friends over dinner and say, "Excuse me, could we change the subject for a second here and talk about my maybe dying?" In support groups, the mention is dicey. If another woman isn't ready to discuss it, you risk deeply disturbing her by bringing it up. As I approached the transplant, though, death was constantly on my mind. I felt like someone whose boss had said, "There's an eighty percent chance we'll be transferring you to Peru within five years, but keep it to yourself."

Laura has no problem talking about Peru, or anything. Will I know what to do if I have to die? I wonder. Umm, millions of people have done it, she muses, and I have to refrain from wise-cracking. "I've seen some beautiful deaths," she adds, making me jump. It takes a while before I can think of death as anything but an aberration or a failure.

Not all our conversations are Andean. Sometimes we compare notes.

"I feel like I've been ejected from my age group," I tell her after a birthday lunch for Claire. Unlike the birthday girl, the other guests only seemed to care about their high-profile careers. I liked my career fine, but felt out of synch; why couldn't they talk about other things, too?

"It's easy to feel like you're divorced from your culture when you've had cancer," she says. "Especially since the culture itself is in the throes of divorce, from illness and death."

Sometimes we just gripe.

"Don't you hate the way they never let you say stress had anything to do with your cancer?" she says in a discussion about official oncological positions.

"I know," I say. "No one would blink if you said you got a cold from working too hard. But if you ever implied stress played any role in your cancer, a support group leader would trample the group to correct you." We'd both investigated the studies. The majority of these hadn't established a conclusive link, a few did implicate stress, and one found that the majority of breast cancer patients thought it had contributed to making them sick, but pooh-poohed them for their belief. "Scientists do not agree," it had quickly added. But Laura and I had seen how far scientists had gotten with the disease. We were going with our gut.

"Yeah," she says. "It's like it's illegal to make any statement that could be misconstrued as meaning a cancer patient caused her own cancer."

If you don't look at what was wrong with your life, you can't change it, one of us invariably remarks at some point during the talk. If I hadn't changed, the other always answers, I bet you for sure I'd be dead by now.

Sometimes we even discuss meditation. Laura introduces me to the concept of the patterned mind. "In India people travel in carts pulled by bullocks, and the carts go along these deep, well-worn grooves," she says, drawing an analogy with consciousness. "People can nod off, so sometimes rocks are placed in the grooves, to jostle them. Many of us are half asleep. The rocks"—life's upsets, obstacles—"keep us awake." Meditation can help you to deal with the rocks, she tells me.

"I've been thinking about how you were brought to the brink of a transplant, then told you were all right," she says. "I'd say that was a pretty big rock."

One Wednesday when she calls, I'm crying. "Bone marrow transplants aren't the magic solution we thought they were," Lambrakis had cautioned me that afternoon. "They only help a small number of women. They're more helpful when there's less bone involvement." He'd paused.

"You have multiple involvement," he'd said.

"But I'm telling you, I have a good feeling about the transplant," I'd argued. He didn't answer.

"Damn him," I say to Laura, so angry I'm blubbering. "I know I'm going to do well, and he won't say it." As focused as an athlete in training, I've reached the eve of the match and the coach has said, "I'm not really sure you're going to make it tomorrow." But what do I want, a doctor who says, "Oh? You know psychically that you're going to be okay? Well, let's just start that transplant now, then, and order the cake for later"? Intuition is crucial to healing, both for doctor and patient. Is it the doctors' fault if protocols and training have purged them of it, if the threat of litigation forces them to give safe responses? I need a pep talk. Lambrakis can only deliver the stats.

"This is a nightmare," Laura says quietly. "You're living in a nightmare." And just the act of someone confirming what I feel brings relief.

"Don't cling to the illusion that this is real," she says, citing Eastern beliefs. "Of course, all of life is an illusion, but this stage of yours is particularly an illusion. You're being tested and will come out stronger, a healer." Laura often refers to tests of strength when we discuss my illness. "You've had a lot of them," she said, and I feel like a circus freak—"Come see the strong man, the lady tattooed by hardship"—but also, secretly, consoled. *This is just a test.*

"I think you're going to make it," she repeatedly says. "I just have that feeling."

Another Wednesday, I ask her about a book. "Have you ever

read *The Battle Against Cancer?* I picked it up last weekend, at Gray-moor." On retreat with a friend at a Franciscan monastery, I'd contributed to the brothers' upkeep with extensive transactions at their bookstore. Thomas Merton's *The Seven Storey Mountain* now tops Mordechai Richler's *Best of American Humor* on the side table.

"I stopped reading illness books that have the words *battle* or *war* in the title," she says. "It's such a militaristic way of looking at it. So long as you think of yourself in battle with cancer, you'll never transcend cancer. You'll always be engaged with it."

Some nights, when there's too much else to talk about, we nearly forget the purpose of the call. "I guess I should ask if you meditated this week," she remembers to inquire before we hang up. Always, unless I've been too high on Dilaudid, I have.

In the living room, dark except for the light of one candle, I fire up a stick of jasmine incense, sit cross-legged on the futon, and close my eyes. Repetition is polish for ritual. Through practice, my meditation and my life acquire luster, even though most nights my mind wanders from the mantra inside of five minutes. It makes a beeline for the office, then creeps into mazes that are so pleasing to explore, I'm reluctant to coax it back. When I do, it bounds out like a puppy, eager to display what it's found. Random thoughts are laid before me: "You have to sift through a lot of mud to find the lotus," I hear the *chi gong* teacher saying. "Music is sustenance," an inner voice observes.

Once, I'm distracted by the sensation of a sweetness so concentrated, it makes me ache. "I've heard people mention that happening," Laura says. "You know what the sweetness supposedly is? Your essence."

The more we talk, and the more I meditate, the more gentled I become. Happiness comes nosing around again. I don't even need to summon or create it. It finds me. In some Hindu sects, happiness is considered the highest form of worship, Laura observes. Gladness courses through me like a prayer.

In this contemplative state, lessons pop out from strange, musty corners. Even chemotherapy becomes a teacher. I'd never thought much about drugs' effect. I'd just assumed they have an immediate impact, then vanish in a day or two. Now I notice how chemo—like divorce, mourning, all things drastic—stays on till it melds with you. For weeks after the injection, you can detect its path as it trails through the body, destroying cells and stamina. Four days later, bone pain. Ten days later, exhaustion. It's been my nature to be reckless, to underestimate the half-lives of all forces, benign and noxious. Taxol forces me to pay attention, to respect the drug's lingering power, to consider what the long-term effects of other substances or experiences might be. "All events are the seeds of future events," it says in one of the Buddhist tracts the corner vegetarian restaurant gives customers to read while they're waiting for their orders. I hope that chemo teaches me to plant wisely.

Through the rest of the summer, my baldness seems like an expression of the internal sanctuary I've come to inhabit, a state of grace that continues through the final Taxol. "Do you have your cap and gown ready?" Joanne e-mails the night before. I do: cap, gown, and wig. I've decided to wear the hairpiece so I can pull it off and toss it into the air at the end.

On the last Taxol Friday, three friends accompany me to the chemo cubicle. They duck out or press up against the walls when my usual nurse, Hindy, comes in to start the drip. The first blast is Benadryl. It makes me floaty. The Taxol, next, turns me red. "Is that air in the line?" Anna says worriedly. "Do you have anything for a sugar buzz?" my friend Joe, who's been passing out chocolates, asks. At noon we make a meal of tofu sandwiches and flaxseed salad, and more chocolates, for dessert. At one o'clock Hindy returns to check the IV.

"Ten more minutes," she announces, dropping the tube.

The plastic bag narrows. Five minutes drag by. Seven, eight. Nine, eleven the bag collapses. My gladness peaks. First my spirits are airborne, then my wig. I am mutant Mary Tyler Moore.

"That's it!" I shout.

"You're done!" my friends yell. We're whooping it up so loudly that if we weren't about to leave, they'd probably have to ask us to.

"Don't take this the wrong way," Hindy says when I find her to say good-bye. "But I hope I never see you again."

"Me, too," I sniffle. "Thank you so much."

This last hurrah's so ebullient, I forget that it doesn't represent the conclusion, but the start. I've got one month off. Then the transplant begins.

Lambrakis calls. They've chosen the date. When we hang up, I log on to the forum. "I'm scheduled for August twenty-fourth," I announce. "I'll go in on a Thursday for the first of two Cytoxans, stay through Sunday, get to be home for two weeks in between. After Cytoxan, they'll bring on the tough stuff: Thiotepa.

"They do transplants outpatient here. Outpatient! I can't believe it. It sounds like the equivalent of a doctor coming to your house and performing open-heart surgery on your living room table. They make you take cabs back and forth to the hospital, and only keep you overnight for chemo and any fevers. It's a way to keep insurance costs down, I'm sure. But my doctor swears the rate of infection isn't any higher than when they put people in isolation. My emotions are high-speed mixed. I'm delighted we're starting, also scared to death."

Applause and assurances pour in. "Great news to know that you're moving ahead!" Joanne writes. "I had two BMTs last year," another woman posts. "Both went well although I had a completely different set of reactions to each. One week after the first I did the Susan Komen 5K race (I'll admit it, I walked). I have had some fatigue and various minor difficulties since but it was worth it for me."

Even the antitransplant crusader weighs in with encouragement, e-mailing an olive branch: "I find myself sharing the hope that the treatment will go really well, that you'll recover very quickly, and that the result will be a complete and lasting remission. We'll all be pulling for you and if wishes and hopes can help, you should get a lot of that kind of assistance, from me no less than the others."

The month off is more like a parole than a reprieve. I thought I'd had every procedure known to oncologists, short of the transplant. But Lambrakis has a couple more surprises in store. He schedules an operation for a second catheter, a loud, embarrassing variety called a Hickman, nothing like the demure bump that's the Mediport. After my head's cleared from the Versed, I see I've got a white, capped hose dangling down my chest, like a backward Chatty Cathy doll. When I tentatively pull on this string to test if the thing's secure, it hurts and makes me say, Fuck.

He gives me a couple of weeks to rest up, then sends me in again, for extraction of the bone marrow that will be reinjected after high-dose. "The bone marrow harvest" is the jolly official name for this step. In between the two surgeries, I spend four mornings at the hospital having a dialysis-like procedure called leukopheresis, in which the boisterous new catheter is used to filter stem cells out of the blood. The stem cells, immune-system concentrates, will also be reinjected later, as further boosters.

Leukopheresis, which takes three hours each visit, is noteworthy for its tedium, nothing more. The only painful aspect is having to listen to dueling television sounds from the small black monitors about the beds. Furniture hucksters squawk about enormous discounts. Remote newscasters cajole bleary-eyed patients and family into *concern* for the state of the world.

Closing my eyes, I try to meditate and overhear a Philippine nurse enthuse about transplants to a research fellow from Spain. "The first one we did, Francesca, eight years ago, she was so sick from cancer when we first saw her," she says. "When she came back six months later, no one could recognize her, she was so healthy." I wait for the punch line. There isn't one. Francesca, she reports, is still alive.

The research fellow stops by my bed. He's shy and curious, polite. Handsome, too. I develop an immediate crush, which deepens to potential love when he says, "There are so many new treatments coming along. Every year, everything changes. The best advice I can give a cancer patient is to just stay alive."

If I make it through the transplant, that's my plan, exactly.

After the second Cytoxan, I forget to sing the river. I'm too distracted and, eventually, too sick. But friends, seen and unseen, circle me, in a chorus. I need to have a fleet of friends, I'd thought sadly when I first found the lump. Now I do.

The week before I entered the hospital, presents arrived in the mail from the forum gang: a book by a 1930s humor writer named Thorne Smith, a good-luck ear cuff in the shape of a lizard. The phone rang continually with offers of help, promises to visit. At the magazine, the editor arranged a lunch to see me off. The staff gave me CDs and cards and a blue velvet hatbox filled with makeup. "It's the good stuff," the beauty editor said.

My parents drove up. We went to the hospital together. My parents waited in the large reception room while I was brought to a back office and given forms to fill out. They came upstairs with me and remarked on the view from my room. "Why, isn't that nice," my father said, even though all that was visible was just rooftops. A nurse came with a blue Gemini pump, and I took charge, loudly and responsibly asking questions. I didn't want my parents to know I felt a little ashamed to have them see me reduced to this.

The nurse popped a needle into the right catheter, and after that, my memories become sketchy. They've been erased less by trauma than by the drugs that were given to do just that.

Sometimes now, a slice from those months comes back: The

night a keening went up outside my hospital room and I crept through the flicker of TV light to see the family spilling out into the hall. "Oh, she was old," the nurse said the next day when I asked who had died, probably to assuage my fear, but making it sound as if old age lessened the importance of death.

The afternoon I couldn't make it to the bathroom fast enough, and the janitor had to come—shades of second-grade shame. The nausea brought on by high-dose chemo was nasty and sharp, even muffled by high counterdoses of an antinausea drug called Nystatin. It made me feel as if I had a pack of rabid dogs under sedation in my stomach.

The way a fever lit into me after the big catheter got infected, causing an emergency and chills so severe my teeth rattled. "You looked like someone in the last stages of AIDS, " Diego says. He was there when the nurses rushed in and wrapped my body in blankets and my head in towels. He wasn't when they raced me down to surgery. "We can't wait to give you the anesthetic," I remember the surgeon saying, although burning with a fever of nearly 103, I may have hallucinated it. "We have to get this thing out." I had no immune system. The germy device could have killed me.

"You were like the walking dead," Diego says.

The zombie memories are mostly lost to my brain. But having brought my laptop with me to the hospital and home again, I do have a kind of epistolary record of those two ghostly months. Rereading cancer forum correspondence from that time, I found that Thiotepa turned my skin brown (*it did?*) and left me weak, but spared me the worst of its side effects—mouth sores so severe that morphine and intravenous feedings must be administered. I discovered that during the first half of the transplant, I employed bravado to quell fear. This was not so bad, I announced to the forum. Just got released from the hospital and went straight to a baby shower, in fact. During the second half, bravado was annealed by the despair of exhaustion. To keep myself going, I would conjure the future—after this was all over, I wanted to cycle through Turkey, I wrote

Joanne—and when I couldn't, when the relentless present bore down too hard, pushing me under, friends stepped in and imagined it for me. "I guarantee you will drink in life once you start getting your health back. This lousy feeling is temporary," a transplant survivor from Ohio e-mailed me in late September, just after the second Cytoxan blast. "In fact, I figure you and I need to have a drink together down the line to celebrate. How about Friday, October 27th, 1 pm EST? You pick the weapon—champagne, beer, etc. We'll toast each and our ability to get on with life."

"All right—you're on," I wrote back from my hospital bed. "I'm going with the best of what I have—herbal tea. It's either that or Nystatin." Others on the forum said they'd join in, and we talked about the power of healing we'd invoke, but at the appointed time, I forgot and slept through it. It didn't matter much, because even if I'd remembered to stay awake for it, the cybertoast would just have made me cry. Everything did, by then.

I'd kept myself pumped up for so long, the crash was inevitable. If I'd allowed myself a wider vision, I might have guessed it was coming. But my sights had had to stay narrowly focused during the preparatory chemo and throughout the transplant. If I'd calculated possible outcomes—thought, for a minute, that the procedure wouldn't work, or that I might survive it only to wish, at times in the aftermath, that I could die—I never would have done it. And I had to. Not that I had to have the transplant—by the time I was eligible, no one was claiming it was the great salvation anymore—but I had to believe something would save me, even if the agent was only fervor and hope. Even if my only real belief was in the belief itself.

Belief precluded foresight. I could not consider what I might have known: That high-dose chemo, like low, takes out inner resources along with white cells, and that high dose, like low, is cumulative. That by the second month, the build of drugs would thicken in my bloodstream, and the promise of completion would be all that was pulling me forward. That I'd be keeping myself going largely on reminders that there would be an end.

The end became everything, but then it arrived, and the end was empty and cold, dead space.

After the fourth blast, I was in for a week before they said it was over, I could go home. This time I didn't whoop or shout. I was too weak to say much when a friend came to meet me. In the cab we were silent. In my lobby I told her I needed a chair. My legs were too unsteady to wait by the elevator. Upstairs the apartment looked windswept and barren. The thin October light reminded me of gruel. My super hadn't turned on the heat yet and I was freezing. For days I couldn't get warm. I ran hot baths, but the tiled bathroom magnified sound in a way that intensified loneliness. I didn't know how dependent I'd become on the hospital's dozy noise till I heard the faucet drip, as loud in the stillness as a gunshot. Hours went by, and no one spoke to me. No one said, "I'm sorry, I just need to check your line" or "Did you remember to collect your urine?" Something bad could have happened. No one would have known.

Sometimes I took three baths a day, one after every nap. But in the tub, I couldn't escape my reflection in the mirrored bathroom door. If I wanted heat, I had to stare at the hairless creature with a tube hanging down her chest, whose skin was a leathery brown. Nothing resembled me except the bottom of my feet.

When the water cooled and made me shiver, I drained some and replaced it with hot. I would cycle heat until my fingertips wrinkled, or until the dripping faucet sounds ricocheted too hard in my depression and drove me back to bed.

Depression made me pliant. I had no bones. "You're a pathetic cancer patient!" I'd berate myself when the force of the floor pushed on my legs and made them soft wax. "You cannot get to the kitchen! You cannot do anything! You are useless!" I hadn't thought to save my fallen hair to make a shirt, but my bald head served fine.

For weeks after the transplant ended, I stayed in this bleak, black place. In fact, I got worse. The horror of what I'd gone through hung in the apartment like gas. The things that happened, the things I saw, I tried to tell all my friends, but they'd seen them, they'd been there with me. They knew, and I was starting to.

By Christmastime my bones had formed again, enough that I could go out. But my nerves stayed shot. Sobs broke over me at home; in grocery lines I trembled. The wrong noise could make me shake. The wrong thought could lead me to contemplate the advantages of death. This end was empty and so was that; the main difference, as far as I could see, was economic. Life required an expenditure of energy. Death didn't, and I had no energy to give.

"You have just gone through a procedure that cost a quarter of a million, in order to stay alive. You cannot spend that kind of money and then kill yourself," I chided myself one day. The absurdity of this position made me smile.

Oh, lovely, I thought, smile widening to a grin. I don't even have the option of suicide.

My legs got stronger. My cell counts rose. By January I started back at work, half days at first, then full. By February I was no longer shouting at cabdrivers who came to quick stops. In early March I bought a yellow duvet, thinking to cover myself in sun. A few weeks later, out on the street, I caught sight of a goofy, vernalated grin on some guy's face and realized that spring was just days off. Soon after, I noticed it: my hair. Okay, I looked like a Chia Pet sprouting fiber optics—no pigmentation yet—but it was there. Two months later, I had a natural buzz cut, a new mountain bike, and plans to cycle through Turkey in the fall. I'd put my money down before I made my first ride, which was a good thing, because the inaugural spin wasn't auspicious. I barely made it from my house to Central Park, a distance of a mile and a half, when I was ready to call for an ambulance.

"You did how many miles?" a friend asked.

"Um, like, three," I said.

"And you're going to do how many on that trip?"

"Up to forty a day," I replied.

"Oh, really," she said, but I didn't respond. I'd learned how to use the future to pull myself into the future. I knew that I'd make it to Turkey, and I knew that Turkey wasn't really the point. That summer I took a place out in Sag Harbor, at the very end of Long Island, and rode ten, then twenty, then thirty miles a day. It was the only way I could think to exhaust the fury and the fight. *The things they'd done*—pump—*the things I'd seen*—

Slam.

EPILOGUE

They found the recurrence three years later, one week after my mother died. "I'm seeing something here, on the adrenals," the doctor running the scan said, and to any cancer patient in her right mind, that would have been cause for panic. But my mind wasn't right, then. It was hazy. My mother had spent the year dying—of lung, liver, heart problems, of everything but Parkinson's. I was numbed by grief too fresh to feel. Cyst, I decided, and in the week before the biopsy, I remained in a state that resembled calm. Cyst. I'd had them before. Cyst, no question, of course— if they scanned anyone every four months, they'd find some weird speck somewhere.

Cyst, but what I didn't consider was the timing. If I'd thought about it, I'd have seen that I'd just gone through the ultimate breakup, a divorce more profound and unyielding than any earthly ending. If my instincts had been firing, I'd have known what was coming. But they weren't. It was the only time that cancer has ever caught me unaware.

When she phoned me at the office, Antonelli sounded composed. The results of the biopsy were in. Just one node. But one node positive. No doubt about it, they were sure. "Listen," she said. "I know we wanted it to be otherwise, but I am not very, very worried. This is not in a life-threatening organ. It's still dependent on hormones—it's more of the same, and as far as prognosis goes, that's excellent." The disease hadn't evolved into a more stubbornly resistant form.

"Of course, recurrences are never good," she said, "but if you're go-ing to have a recurrence, you're having it in the best possible way."

But when she phoned my home machine, immediately after we'd hung up, her voice was sorrowful and slow. "I'm calling you now as your dear, dear friend," the message on the tape began. "I am so sorry that I had to give you this news at a time like this. But, you know, I wanted to tell you something I truly, truly believe. You have triumphed in every battle in the past. I have no doubt whatsoever that you will triumph again."

Despite her rousing vote of confidence, I was afraid she sounded as stunned as I felt.

All afternoon I made arrangements—with a pharmacy, to pick up Cytadren; I was going back on the hormone that had trounced the illness before. With Claire, Anna, all my close friends; no way, this time, would I hole up alone. With my boss, for a two-month leave to concentrate on alternative treatments. "We'll do whatever you need," she said, as quickly as she had the first time I'd sat before her and said, "It's, um, it's back." Before I packed it in for the night, I put in one more call, to Rick Harri-son, the brilliant Tennessee oncologist from the cancer forum. I wasn't really looking for a second opinion; my trust in Antonelli was complete. More, I wanted a second reassurance.

"Do you have children?" Harrison asked after I'd filled him in at length on my history, the recent relapse, and my concern that I'd be a fool to be optimistic.

"No," I said. Was he suggesting I make provisions?

"Oh. Well—I was going to say, Don't worry, you'll see your grand-children. But no kids? Okay. Then, in that case, here's my advice to you: Buy the radial tires."

During the next two months, I drank sharp concoctions of carrot, garlic, and cabbage juice. I started on Tibetan herbs. I had injections of

Pamidronate, a drug that caused fevers but could help prevent a second spread to the bones. I meditated. I ran. I imagined healing rays of light softening the stiff, crusty node. I was sure, by the time I went for the second scan, that I was kicking that cancer's ass.

"Stable," Antonelli said after the technicians reported back. "I know you wanted it to shrink, but stable is eighty percent good. The cancer hasn't grown, and that means the Cytadren is working. If it weren't, the tumor would have grown." Besides, she said, two months might be a little early to test a hormone's effect. Why didn't we schedule another scan for, say, two months on, see what we found then?

"Stable," she said two months and two days later. "Stable, but this is not a bad result. In fact, I mean it: It makes me happy. Stable is not what you were after, but I promise you, stable is good."

I must not have sounded as if I shared her rosy vision, because when I returned home that night, I found a message on the machine.

"I wanted to explain why I said I was happy," Antonelli said. "I wasn't just telling you that. First of all, there is a possibility that what we're seeing here is just a scar. It may be the cancer is gone, and if you continue stable, we can find a way to test and see if that's true. But even if the disease is still there, stable is very good."

For one thing, she reminded me, so many new treatments are available or in development, oncologists now consider metastatic breast cancer a chronic illness. Like diabetes, is how they often put it. "People have flare-ups and then they get better," she said. "They continue to lead lives."

For another, she said, my disease had responded to everything they'd thrown at it so far. It was weak and slow and it had gone away in the past, with treatment. With treatment, it would almost certainly go away again. "I know you wanted it to disappear," she said. "But maybe this is better. Cancer that goes away fast comes back fast."

With a slow kind, especially, they could treat it for a very long time, and that's what some oncologists meant when they declared metastatic breast cancer a curable disease. Not that they could get rid of it for good. Yet. But they could often rout it for extended periods, and when it came *back, rout it again. Or they could keep it in stasis, impotent and checked. Antonelli had many patients who'd been walking around stable for years and years.*

"The fact that you keep coming back stable is a really encouraging sign," she said. "Really," she said. "It's all good news."

ron kurtz

As a gay man and the adult child of a Holocaust survivor, Ron Kurtz touches on the role of shared experience as a means of healing—and the difficulty in
waiting for the right moment for it to occur.

our sunday conversation

It never really occurred to me that my father had any kind of an accent until I moved away to college and spoke to him by phone once every few weeks. Before then it was just something I had learned to live with, and took for granted, like the way he used to play poker with his friends in our kitchen most Monday nights.

My father's poker friends were small, brutish-looking men with wiry clumps of hair bristling from their ears. They spoke in loud, hysterical voices, almost like women, and in between, dealers took long breaks. I used to duck inside before bedtime, when no one was watching, to grab a handful of potato chips. As I spied on them from behind the kitchen counter they shifted nervously in their chairs, passed around cigars, and rolled up their shirtsleeves to reveal their tattoos. They all had nearly identical tattoos.

When I was five or six, I remember asking my mother about the row of numbers scrawled into my father's skin. "What is that?" She stood over me, toweling my hair after my Tuesday night bath. I used to think it was some sort of code, like the pieces of a treasure map someone had put there. I can't really remember how she answered except to say he had once been a prisoner, a response that did nothing to satisfy my curiosity. All I knew was that it meant something bad. I used to think, even hope, that maybe my father had gone to jail. Maybe all of his friends, his poker buddies, once shared the same cell. Maybe they were bank robbers or something worse.

My father had always been a mysterious figure. He worked long hours and always came home late, as I was getting ready for bed. He used to come into my room and brush his face against mine. His day's growth of whiskers was rough against my smooth mouth and cheeks. I idolized him. He resembled Sean Connery with his dark hair, thick shoulders, and hairy chest. I used to stand in the bathroom mirror with the door locked and study my thin, prepubescent body for something physical—like some chest hair of my own—that would connect me to him.

One of my earliest childhood memories is of buying a temporary tattoo from a candy machine at the local supermarket and pasting it to my forearm in the exact same place as my father wore his. When I got home, I made the mistake of showing it to my mother. A terrible look came across her face. She grabbed me by the wrist and marched me into the bathroom. I was afraid she was going to slap me, but instead she forced me to scrub it off, using an old washcloth and soap, until I started to cry. She made me promise never to do anything so foolish again. My father never saw it.

Now I'm thirty-seven and my father is seventy. He has recently retired, having sold the only thing that ever really mattered to him, a small men's clothing store he owned and managed for thirty years. He calls me every Sunday morning from the new house he's bought on a small lake outside Detroit. He doesn't know what to do with himself. He's never had any hobbies or interests except his store. He calls me, not my two older brothers, because they're married and have lives of their own, settled in California with thriving medical practices, mortgages, wives, and three children apiece.

He calls me because he's depressed and perhaps even lonely. Although he's been married to his second wife for the past seventeen years—a woman he met six months after my mother died—she has her own life, with grown-up children and grandchildren, her own set of problems.

He finds it easier to talk to me because I understand that his life has not turned out the way he wanted it to. He calls because he knows I'll listen. My life is still unsettled, and he hopes maybe he can talk some sense into me. He calls because he knows I still need him.

"You have to write yourself a check for the rent," he reminds me at the beginning of each month. "Though I know you can't afford it. Not on your salary."

Until recently, my father had gotten into the habit of sending me money each month to cover my expenses. I took the money reluctantly and told him not to send me anything more. To me, this monthly check was a kind of emotional blackmail. It reminded me that I was still a child, incapable of taking care of myself.

To understand my father one must know that his life's philosophy was forged in Europe during the Holocaust. A Polish Jew, born in Lodz, my father lost much of his family, including his mother and only sister when the Nazis began liquidating the ghetto. His father died of tuberculosis shortly before the war. The Germans forced my father from one prison camp to the next, marching several hundred miles at a time in freezing snow. He's told me stories about someone he knew, a next-door neighbor, or family friend, who fell exhausted into the snow to rest and in the morning never got up again. He carries this experience with him still, a tremendous weight that never seems to lift even when he smiles.

"Nothing excites me," my father tells me. "I go into the garden out back and plant a few flowers, perennials or something, and I'm tired. All I want to do is come inside and rest."

"You should take a class," I tell him. "Or develop an interest. Tony Curtis didn't start painting until he was your age, and now look at him. He's embarked on a whole new career."

"Ach," my father says, and I can see him making a sour face into the phone, waving off such a notion. "Who cares about Tony Curtis? He was such a great actor?"

"Well, you have to do something. You're driving yourself crazy."

My father spends his afternoons at the local Jewish Community Center with all the other retirees, many of whom are survivors like himself, old men in their sixties and seventies who sit in the steam room, *shvitzing* and complaining about their kids. Here he's in his

element. No one laughs at his theories or rolls his eyes when he offers advice. Not like his kids. These people all have similar tales of
woe about sons or daughters who refuse to get married or choose a
bad relationship and get divorced or make foolish business decisions
and go broke.

It's mainly for this reason, my fear of being made into yet another anecdote of a good son "gone bad," that I tell my father very
little about my life. This hasn't stopped him, however, from telling
me about the trouble he has sleeping at night because he's too busy
worrying about my future and whether I'll ever find a career. When
I was laid off four years ago from my last job in publishing, I didn't
say anything to him about it for several months.

"You should have a profession," he told me the last time he
called. "That's your problem. Your brothers went to school and studied medicine. You went to school and studied literature. That's not
a profession." For my father's generation, the question is never
whether the glass is half full or half empty. But rather, where did
this water come from? Is it even safe to drink?

The first time I left a particularly stressful work situation, I
made the mistake of telling him all about it. I spent the rest of our
conversation consoling him, reassuring him that a better job was
waiting down the road and that it was only a matter of time before
I found it.

Not that my father doesn't have reason to be concerned. Since
moving to New York ten years ago, I've held one editorial position
after another, never really getting ahead due in part to bad luck: a
string of crazy bosses, corporate downsizing, and restructuring. At
least that's the official reason. In truth, it may have something more
to do with my fear of allowing myself to get stuck in a job I don't
really want when all I really want to do is write.

Stand up to him, my friends say. Tell him who you are and that
what you do is none of his business. But he's my father, I answer
back. He's suffered all his life. How much more pain can I give

him? Or for that matter, how much more pain can I take myself, telling him the truth and having to live with the consequences of my decision?

That I've managed to tell him I've been volunteering for several AIDS service organizations over the past several years, including Gay Men's Health Crisis, seems to me a victory of sorts. At least he's stopped asking whether there are any women in my life. That I haven't said anything more is a testament to how much my father is able to accept and understand.

The last time I visited him he found me sitting in his living room watching an old television documentary from the eighties, about the impact of the AIDS epidemic on the population of San Francisco. They interviewed Randy Shilts, still handsome and very much alive, with his thick mop of curly black hair and quick, intelligent eyes magnified behind owl-framed glasses. The film kept cutting back and forth between Randy and footage of a gay man dying in his hospital bed, his jaundiced eyes shallow and sunken into his face, his lips a blue, trembling line.

"You help these people?" my father said, indicating the screen. "You go into their homes and help them?"

"Sometimes I'll walk this guy's dog. Buy him groceries, or help clean up his apartment."

"Are all of them this sick?" he said.

"Sometimes worse."

"Well, whatever you do," he said, "if they offer you something to eat, don't take it."

Although the concern registered in his eyes, I didn't know how to respond, or what to say next.

"You're being ridiculous," I finally said, thinking about all the HIV-positive boyfriends I've had and all the things he wouldn't want to know about that have gone into my mouth.

My father's apparent ignorance often disturbs and vexes me. He has known what it is to load the bodies of the dead onto carts for mass burial and has had most of his molars rot and fall from his mouth due to malnutrition. But still, his experiences have not necessarily given him any greater insight into the human condition. If anything, they have made him even more intolerant. For my father, the world has been roughly divided into one of victims and victimizers, where there is a kind of hierarchy placed on human suffering in which all the various social injustices visited upon the Jews take precedence over the hurt and injustices experienced by others. He has no patience for the plight of Vietnam vets and all their rallying to be heard ("crybabies," he calls them) and is indignant about the poverty, crime, and drug abuse of the inner-city *shvartze* (his word, not mine). On occasion, I have even seen him smile in almost sadistic pleasure at the images of war-torn Bosnia flashing across his TV screen. "Those anti-Semitic bastards," he's told me, "are finally getting what they deserve."

I would like to think that being gay and being the adult child of a Holocaust survivor have given me a more profound understanding of the sufferings of others. After all, gay men and lesbians are America's last minority and as such are still considered "socially acceptable" to despise. Being the adult child of a Holocaust survivor has meant something that many of my friends who have survived the AIDS epidemic still can't quite understand; it's meant carrying a large part of my father deep inside me. I can sometimes feel the weight of his history and the pain he's suffered—a kind of burden I can't escape even if I wanted to.

I may not remember the precise moment when all the obvious pieces fell into place, when I first came to realize that my father had lived through a moment in history that most have only read about in books, but I can still recall the giddy excitement of lying on my stomach in my family's den, perched in front of our color TV, watching Ron Ely swinging half naked through the trees, and trying to hide from my brothers the erection growing through a hole in my pajamas.

At eight years old, I knew I was different. When an older cousin of mine came out of the closet it all started to make sense. I felt a strange kind of relief in knowing I was not alone. Relief quickly turned to shame when, soon after his announcement, my cousin was ostracized from our family.

My father had always said there was something funny about Kenny, and he refused to let any of us use the word *queer* again. "I never liked that word," he said.

Perhaps I'm selling my father short. I know he loves me. But he's from a different time and culture, when such things as illness and death, and—certainly—homosexuality were considered too shameful for discussion and were conveniently ignored.

I became a conspirator in my parents' house, privy to all the jokes and comments my brothers made behind our cousin's back, making many of these same comments myself for fear of being discovered. I turned all of my brothers' hatred inside and directed it against myself. Throughout junior high, I remember being conscious of the way I walked down the hallway and of how I looked carrying my books at my side.

Years later, after completing my graduate studies, I moved to New York, and like so many other gay men who came to the City seeking their fame and good fortune, I had yet to discover my place in the world and fell into a series of dizzying relationships with men who fed my damaged self-esteem. They were all of a certain type: young and ambitious, with a rakish charm and the inability to commit to anything long term. After more than six months of this, I gave up and began volunteering for the AIDS community. It was cheaper than dating and almost less traumatic.

The son of an old family friend invited me to join his support group, which met in the basement of a synagogue near Gramercy Park. I attended these meetings curious to discover what they might teach me about myself. All of their members, both men and women, were the adult children of Holocaust survivors.

While they had the usual complaints adult children have about their parents—their parents never listened, their parents never gave them the emotional support they needed or said nice things in front of their friends—they also talked about the sense they shared of feeling disconnected from some important aspect of their parents' lives. I heard one woman say it was like living with some shameful secret that everyone knew about but never discussed. Whenever someone in her family had the nerve to ask what had really happened to Aunt Ruth or Uncle Leon, an awkward silence filled the room.

As the only gay member of this group, I knew all about "shameful secrets," especially when dealing with older aunts or cousins who wanted to know why I wasn't settled down or hadn't yet married. At the same time, I could relate to the isolation the others expressed. Friends of mine could point to family pictures on the wall. We had no pictures of my father's family on our walls. There was nothing personal to connect us to him. Nothing but a deep sense of loss and discomfort whenever any of us, my brothers or my mother, asked him something directly about himself.

And so, every Sunday morning he calls to tell me that he has nothing more to do. He complains that whenever he calls my brothers' families in California no one ever makes time for him. "They're always off running around," he says. "Going, going, going. Taking the boys to baseball practice, and the girls to tennis and ballet. You guys were never so busy growing up." His voice takes on a wounded, almost petulant tone.

Perhaps it's because my father lost so much of his own family when he was young that he expects my brothers, their wives and children, to be more closely connected, to give him back something he's lost or never really had. But, growing up, my father had never been much of a physical presence in our lives. He never went to my brothers' football games, and never attended any of my high school productions. We never tossed a ball around in the backyard or went on fishing or camping trips. I never learned how to play the sports he enjoyed, like soccer. The first time my brothers and I got to know him was when we were old enough to work for him at his store. We dusted off the men's suits on the racks, priced the jeans and dress shirts, helped him set up the outside tables, and managed the summer's sidewalk sales, making sure nothing was stolen.

My father and I became closer shortly before my mother died, when I returned home from college to help him take care of her. My brothers were just getting started in their own lives, both of them having recently married. One of them was already in California. The other had a baby girl on the way, my parents' first grandchild.

I helped my mother get dressed in the mornings, made her hot cereal and protein milkshakes. In the afternoons we went for long walks around the block; sometimes she stopped to catch her breath, her fingers pressed into my arm. She asked me why the chemotherapy wasn't making her feel any better. I lied to her. Told her something stupid like she was getting better all the time. She just didn't know it yet. We never told her she was dying. It was my father's decision. He was afraid she might give up hope.

After the funeral I stayed on in Detroit until February. My father and I went to synagogue every Friday night for services. We recited the mourner's Kaddish so many times that we eventually learned it by heart.

One particular evening, while we walked home through the snow, still wearing our dress shoes, I asked him whether he ever believed in God, or felt God's presence with him in the camps.

"I felt something," he told me. "But it was against us."

Years later when I asked him to explain what he had felt in greater detail, he couldn't seem to remember or to confirm anything more about it. It left me with the uneasy feeling that perhaps our conversation had never really happened, that his response had been a fabrication on my part, something I had made up as a desperate attempt to connect.

My father doesn't talk much about his childhood, what was taken from him during the war. "What's past is past," he likes to say. But no matter how many times I may argue or tell him that it is our past that shapes us and makes us who we are, he refuses to listen. My father says he keeps his silence to protect us. "But from what?" I've asked him. He never answers, and I can only guess at the horrors he's witnessed.

All that I've been able to gather, to hold on to, comes in small pieces of information offered randomly. Like the time when he was in the hospital for exploratory surgery. Maybe he thought he'd never pull through, or maybe it was because he had all of his sons gathered around him, but he was overcome with emotion. He told us more about his experiences than I can remember him ever telling us before.

He told us what had happened after he and his uncle Max were boarded on the train for Auschwitz. He told us how they were placed in two separate lines. My father was only fourteen or fifteen years old and refused to be taken from his uncle. He was carrying their bread, which his aunt had sewn into the lining of his coat. Another worker, perhaps a Jew, grabbed my father by the collar and forced him back into his original place in line.

"You stay where you're put," this worker said. He never saw his uncle again.

At such moments, the present world seems to stop and you can almost see my father straining to touch something elusive and intangible, like the frosted edges of a photograph lying at the bottom of a tray of chemicals, the images shimmering ghostlike and powerful.

I talk to him now in my cramped studio apartment, twisting the phone cord between my fingers, the rain beating against the windows. It's Memorial Day weekend, and I've chosen to stay here because all my friends have gone away, and the city is quiet. I pull open the blinds and see into my neighbor's living room in the next building, where the walls are all painted white, where there is expensive track lighting and brightly colored art tastefully arranged. It's the kind of apartment I know my father wishes for me.

I sit on my sagging futon mattress, the cheap metal frame bent and straining beneath my weight. The *Sunday Times* from two weeks ago lies scattered across the floor. There are books and magazines everywhere, falling off the shelves, or stacked in piles at the foot of my bed. I'm watching a nature special on TV, with the sound off, about how baby cougars once grown are never allowed to return to their nest.

Before my father has a chance to speak I can feel the tremendous sadness stirring on his end of the line.

After all these years, it is through this sadness that we have finally managed to connect.

And yet, I still wait with a certain expectation that he will give me back something to hold on to. That he will be able to provide me with the necessary thing I lack: a deeper understanding that illuminates his experiences, and my own. But lately, my father has begun to sound like any other man his age. He's achieved a kind of complacency about the way things are, no matter how miserable. It is a complacency that has cheated me from learning anything more.

He clears his throat and tells me he's getting older. He says he's depressed. He's been waking every morning to find a familiar stiffness creeping into his legs.

I share his frustration. This nameless anxiety that binds us. This weight that never seems to shift.

My father sighs.

I just nod my head and listen to him breathing. His eyes blink behind thick folds of skin.

"I'm gay," I want to tell him. "I'm gay, and I'm still your son."

The silence on his end is deafening, a terrible roar.

But still it is something. A place to begin.

tom sleigh

"The Incurables" is simultaneously accurate and informative, yet electrified with dream and fantasy. Sleigh's remarkable achievement is in how the jarring details of his life help illuminate his erudite philosophical ruminations.

the incurables

Fifteen years ago, in a place that now seems less likely than anything I could make up, I find myself sitting in a room in a Mexican clinic that treats patients on whom conventional medicine had given up. In other rooms there are other patients, some of them within days or weeks of their deaths. Perhaps to call it a "clinic" is too grand. The fact is, we have retreated to a converted motel—in better days, it served as a retreat for Hollywood stars like Gloria Swanson and Dorothy Lamour. At least that's the myth we trade among ourselves, compensating for the cracked ceilings and walls in our rooms, the chipped and dirty swimming pool, the haphazard palm trees, and the overgrown bougainvillea that clings to the faded whitewashed wall that surrounds the clinic grounds.

Removed from the world, we drink specially prepared juices each hour for fourteen hours, we eat vegetarian meals, we try to detoxify our bodies with frequent enemas. At the end of our first week, if the treatment is working, our immune systems will react with astonishing ferocity: our organs and tissues will begin dumping toxins into our bloodstreams, the cancer patients' tumors will start to dissolve. The result of all this purifying activity, in which the body supposedly gears up to heal itself, is high fever, nausea, acute pain in the joints as calcium deposits break down, foul odors, sweats, sudden intense chills, even mild forms of mental disturbance and psychosis. The challenge is to stay ahead of the flood of poisons.

Only the fear of imminent death could make anyone stick to this regimen. Six, seven, or more enemas a day—the treatment seems lunatic fringe at best. But what can we do? Fasting, visualization, macrobiotics, laetrile, wheat grass juice—we've read the literature, we've given these other alternatives a try. And still we're sick, our doctors still tell us there's nothing they can do. As our chances for getting well diminish, as pain or weakness turns us more and more inward, the only force turning us back toward the world is hope.

Having lived with a chronic blood disease for close to twenty years, I've become acquainted with the mercurial shiftings of hope. Hope is my ally when my health starts to decline, convincing me that I can raise myself up; but hope is equally my tormentor: in a good stretch of health, hope can lull me into thinking that my life is more or less normal—until the inevitable downswing, when hope seems merely self-delusion.

My illness is as rare as it is unpronounceable: "paroxysmal nocturnal hemoglobinuria"—which in simple English means "blood in your urine at night." The first time I noticed it was on a dank, hot, Baltimore spring morning a few months after I'd turned twenty-two. To keep my fear in check, I walked the floor of my apartment a few items, halting now and then at the window to look down at a plane tree that was just beginning to leaf out above the Dumpster in the alley. I managed to convince myself that the blood lazily diffusing in the toilet water was only a fluke of biochemistry—a verdict that the various doctors I consulted with over the next three years tended to agree with. None of them came remotely close to making the right diagnosis—a fact I don't hold against them. There are so few cases that most doctors, including blood specialists, have never actually seen a walking, talking PNH patient.

The disease (*my* disease, I should say) has no known precipitating cause—but somehow a gene that should make a protective protein on the membrane wall of a red blood cell has gotten switched off. So when I get an infection or if I'm overtired, my oxygen-carrying red blood cells break down abnormally fast. In fact, if I contract a particularly fierce fever, my red cells begin to explode so quickly in my bloodstream that unless I get to a hospital, I can die—from a loss of blood, from blood clots, from heart attack. And those are only the acute dangers: in the long term my disease can develop into leukemia, or my bone marrow can give out altogether—what the Merck Manual calls "aplastic anemia." But when my blood count is stable, I take an almost macho pride in my body's ability to adjust: a normal person reading this essay would probably faint in his chair and be in serious need of a transfusion if his red cell count began to plummet to the level that I now consider "healthy."

In these good periods, as if my illness were a demon lover, my muscles flex and bend: I try to appease my illness with feats of strength and endurance, to blind and nullify it by swimming and hiking and taking long walks.

But then, as always, comes the crash—I get a fever, my blood count starts to dive, hope neutralizes to fear by fueling what I know is the excessive intensity of my fantasy life: as if to counter my lack of physical vitality, my daydreams grow wildly involuted. While the skeptic in me scoffs, I dream up obscure and mystical compensations for the knowledge that sooner, rather than later, my body will fail me.

The hope that my death can mean something, mean something not just to my intimates but to the world at large, drives me in the most shameless and childish way to concoct extravagant, even grandiose fantasies. The more elaborate the fantasy, the graver the circumstance: snowed in beneath hospital sheets, as I wave good-bye to my construction worker roommate (whose blood count had inexplicably gone to the level *up* to which I'm waiting to be transfused), the orderly slides me out of bed onto the green, plastic-pillowed trolley and wheels me off to X ray. I'm to undergo a scan for clots in my lungs. While I breathe in the radioactive gas that will illuminate my lung tissue, I fight back my fear of death with a fantasy in which I embrace death: the plastic mask erasing my features, suddenly I'm hectoring and stoical, casually unconcerned by the approach of my impending execution. I spend my final hours convincing my closest friends that the soul is imperishable . . . without a tremor, I drink off the fatal hemlock that my weeping jailer prepares for me. Unlikely or laughable as it seems, I'm reenacting Socrates' state-ordered suicide, my so-called crime to incite free thinking in the young. The fact that I'm terminally ill, and my death is less a sacrifice on the altar of free thought than it appears, is my closely guarded secret.

In the *Phaedo,* the dialogue by Plato that recounts Socrates' death and his attempt to prove the immortality of the soul, I sense beneath his manner of disinterested, logical argument wild swings of hope and fear: hope that death will reveal the ultimate truth, fear that all death means is that one's heart stops beating. How confident the philosopher seems in his talk of mind disencumbered of body, pure, immortal mind! Yet beneath the deliberate cool with which he elucidates the doctrine of the divine, eternal forms, showing how "Beauty and Goodness possess a most real and absolute existence," I sense in his willingness to take the poison something murkily self-destructive, almost suicidal. At the same time, his conviction that the soul is immortal is more than a little self-interested: as his proofs elaborately unravel into counterproofs, he demonstrates not only the immortality of the Soul, but of his soul in particular. But these spookily contradictory motives aren't simply the product of an unacknowledged death wish or a maniacally hopeful need to reassure himself of his own indestructibility—the philosopher seems equally intent on comforting his followers. Tenderly stroking the head of Phaedo, Socrates asks his young friend if he intends to cut his hair tomorrow as a sign of mourning. When the heartbroken Phaedo laconically replies, "Yes, Socrates, I suppose I will," the philosopher jokes that if his arguments fail, both of them will have to shave their heads today.

What I find most moving and troubling about this dialogue is the moment of Socrates' death, when he pits his own hope for immortality against the implicitly skeptical method of his argument. Each time he establishes the soul's indestructibility, he encourages his followers to contradict him, poke holes in his conclusions until they are completely satisfied that the case has been proven. At last all doubts are vanquished, his followers accept his reasons; his approaching death and his eerily hopeful embrace of it are in precarious balance.

But now my fantasy takes over, the soul of Socrates inhabits my lungs, lips, teeth, tongue that have been arguing against the body as frail, corrupt—while the hemlock numbs my flesh, my friends feel my feet, ankles, knees, thighs to keep track of how far up my body the chill of the hemlock has progressed. My philosophical abstractions, my denigration of my own flesh are entirely forgotten before the mystery of the dying body. The elaborate dance of my intellect can't distract me or my friends from the sorrow and fascination of flesh passing away, flesh that means me, my hand stroking my friend's hair. My vision is blurring . . . to spare my friends the sight of my face, I've drawn a cloth over my head. But now a sacrifice that I've overlooked to Asclepius, the divine healer, keeps nagging at me: I uncover my face and fixing my eyes on Crito, the friend I most trust, I tell him, "Crito, we owe a cock to Asclepius. Make sure the debt is paid." When he assures me it will be done, I—.

But here the fantasy comes to a full stop. I'm no longer Socrates; his soul has passed out of my flesh . . . my fantasy gives way to the fact that for almost twenty years, I've anticipated daily, whether consciously or not, the moment of my death. . . . The fact of my death, my *real* death, is a scalpel that cuts through tissues of ego and daydream: in another starker vision of the end, I see my body shiver a little while my lungs stop breathing. But my mind can't rest there, death is too reductive, it can't keep hope from spurring on my imagination: now Hermes appears and leads my soul flittering like a bat to the underworld. The soul of my dead father comes winging up to me, shrilling in a frequency I don't yet understand—except for the strange vibration of *hope,* the lone syllable in the language of the dead that is anything like the language of the lives of earth.

. . .

My father comes to me in a dream. His fur is white, his antlers branch above him, his muzzle is elongated, his nostrils quiveringly suspicious. His eyes see me but don't see me as he lowers his head to drink. The water drips from his jaws when he raises his head again, and now his eyes, which before were liquid, uncomprehending, wholly animal, stare back at me with human recognition. He seems to know me, but he himself—I can't tell what he's feeling or thinking. He takes a step toward me and as I put my hand out to touch his fur, his head jerks back, and he looks at me warily—but then allows me to put my arm around his neck, blood-warm, his fur more bristly than it looks. I feel joy to have him next to me, his fur, his muscled legs, the ridge of his long backbone—but in the next moments he flattens into two dimensions, and I realize that I'm looking at a mosaic. A voice that I can't locate says, "Stop, just stop it!" when I wake a moment later, I can tell that my health, which has been poor for the past few days, is better, magically better, and that the renewed strength I feel in my arms, and especially in my legs, has something to do with my dream.

In A.D. 174 Pausanias, the Greek travel writer, visited Epidaurus in southern Greece, the center of the cult of Asclepius. He tells us that Asclepius's father is Apollo, god of medicine, music, light, and prophecy while his mother, Coronis, is mortal. The polarity of an immortal father and mortal mother underscores the ups and downs of the god's fortunes. In one story of his birth, his mother leaves him to die on a mountain (ironically named Mount Nipple), while in another he is snatched by Hermes from his dead mother's womb just as the flames of her funeral pyre engulf her. Entrusted by Apollo to Chiron, the wise centaur, for his education, Asclepius brings the healing arts to such perfection that the gods of the underworld complain that they are cheated of their dead—and so Zeus incinerates Asclepius with a thunderbolt. But the cult of Asclepius springs up all over Greece: Pausanias describes the god's many statues as being made of ivory and gold. The god is seated and a dog lies next to him. One hand grasps a staff, the other is held above the head of a serpent. As the god's birthplace, Epidaurus becomes one of the healing centers of the ancient world.

In Asclepius's wild oscillations of fortune—his exposure on the mountain, his rescue from his mother's funeral pyre, his ability to raise the dead, for which he himself is put to death—I perceive the force of human ingenuity struggling against the brute fact of death: Asclepius's brushes with death and his miraculous escapes seem an emblem of the human mind faced with its own mortality as it ricochets between hope and despair.

What in Epidaurus was called the Hieron, or sacred precinct, of Asclepius, finds its counterpart in the clinic dining room. This is the sacred space of our hope to get well. To an outsider, in our short-sleeved shirts and sandals we look as casual as tourists on a Mexican holiday. But the pallid woman who sits across from me, who seems to labor to bring her spoon up to her lips, the hoarsely breathing man next to me whose skin is more jaundiced than tan, concentrate on their food with fanatical intensity. In our sect of the sick, in which we secretly speculate on the ones among us who are too far gone to make it, our cardinal rule is to convince each other and ourselves that health can't be too far away. As we sit eating at the battered wooden table, novitiates like myself glean knowledge from the old hands:

"Had your first fever?"

"No, it hasn't hit me yet."

"Mine lasted about four days—one hundred four degrees, nausea, the works. The docs here are right about the peppermint tea. It washes out your stomach real good. And you should do double duty with the enemas. It really helps to knock the fever down."

I stare into an unseasoned soup of potatoes, onions, and leeks. My ears fill with the hum of an industrial juicer reducing crates and crates of kale, celery, beet tops, apples, carrots to a messy pulp squeezed by a hydraulic press into the elixirs we drink. All of us smell subtly of the Vaseline we grease our enema tubes with.

"Are you doing full-strength coffee enemas?"

"No, they told me to try tea for a while—just to go easy, at first."

To traditional practitioners of medicine, all this sounds crackpot—a hypermoralized quackery that stresses "cleansing," an almost ritualized regulation of eating habits and bodily evacuations that is reminiscent of certain practices of ancient mystery religions that stress the need for purification and rebirth: initiates into Mithraism were placed into a pit where the blood of a sacrificed bull streamed down on them from above, washing them clean of their sinful past lives; like Socrates' devotees, Pythagoras's followers believed in the transmigration of the soul; that it passed from body to body until it became so pure that it was released from the cycle of death and rebirth; Orphic cults prescribed ascetic practices to believers; no beans, no flesh, the wearing of certain kinds of clothes. Such ancient rites and disciplines seem oddball at best, akin in certain respects to the healing cult of the Virgin Mary at Lourdes. Mystical mummery, faith healing, it all sounds pretty dubious . . . but I wasn't going to discount the miracle that could cure me!

In the sacred groves of Asclepius stretched a long, covered colonnade where patients consulting the god would sleep, see certain visions in dreams, and come forth cured the next morning. Did the dream of my father as a stag have a clinically measurable effect on the sudden improvement in my health? The temptation to link my dream with the therapeutic power of mental suggestion is hard to resist—especially when doctors can accurately describe the biochemical chain reactions that make me feel sick, but offer nothing concrete in the way of a cure . . . except for a potentially risky bone marrow transplant. High doses of radiation and chemotherapy to wipe out my bone marrow mean that I would have to live in hygienic isolation from infection. Temporarily without an immune system until the new marrow infused into me can take hold, I would be defenseless against the most innocuous of microbes.

When I contemplate undergoing a marrow transplant, I begin to allegorize the stages of marrow transplantation into a quasi-mystical passage from disease to health. First, the ritual ablution, in which my sinful marrow is destroyed; through an intravenous needle, Cytoxan swirls into my bloodstream, or I lie on the X-ray table absorbing megadoses of radiation. Then, in a germ-free plastic tent, I'm kept in isolation from the world's manifold pollution: utterly nauseous and wiped out in my high-tech chrysalis, I pass through the stages of my rebirth: my clean new marrow is IV'd into my veins and sucked up by the hollows of my bones; gradually, over a week or two of obsessive monitoring and blood tests, my new marrow cells proliferate and take hold . . . and if all goes well . . . if the graft is successful and my defective red blood cells don't return . . . if, during the month or so of my sojourn in this germicidal void, I've successfully avoided pneumonia and other life-threatening infections . . . then—at last!—my day of deliverance arrives: I take off my surgical mask, I leave my tent; through the hospital's automatic doors I step out into the microbe-infested air, I reenter the world of temptation and risk.

Of course, a bone marrow transplant ought not to be mystified; it isn't an allegory of sin and salvation, of spiritual death and rebirth. But the relatively neutral phrase, "bone marrow transplant"—nothing in the term hints at how extreme the treatment is. Of course, that neutrality buffers me from the knowledge that my doctors must deliberately bring me close to death as part of my cure: not quite as theatrical as being washed in bull's blood, but a whole lot riskier. Who can blame me for indulging in a little mythmaking? Even if I don't succumb to infection while my new marrow is grafting, I'm still subject to the irony that to make me well is to make me ill; released from the hospital, in full possession of my new health, I'm haunted by my treatment's future consequences: just what are the long-term effects of high doses of radiation and chemotherapy?

. . .

I'm lying on a doctor's examining table. My neck is crooked at a strange angle to the pillow, almost as if it were broken. I try to turn my head so that my neck is no longer twisted, but I'm so exhausted that I can't even muster the strength to lift my head off the pillow. Now I hear a faint rustling sound and see water begin to seep around the edges of the table, advancing slowly the way the tide in a quiet bay advances. And then I realize that the room is suspended like a bubble of breath in the depths of the ocean. The water seeps in more quickly now, and I'm beginning to feel desperate: I can't keep the water out unless I get up from the table, but I'm so worn out I can't even lift my head.

In one case recorded at Epidaurus, a sleeping patient woke to find the spearhead embedded in his jaw miraculously extracted and placed in his hand. And there are other accounts where hysterical or similar afflictions were cured by the influence of imagination or sudden emotion. True or not, these stories were much like the stories we told each other over meals at the clinic. To an outsider, there isn't much spiritual uplift in these tales. In fact, in our relish to recount the history of our own bodily functions, we sound a little like the sinners in Dante's hell as they eagerly recount the history of their sins:

"My hands and feet began to sweat this afternoon in the weirdest way. But when they stopped, the headache I'd had all afternoon was gone."

"I was nauseous for a while this morning until I vomited up a lot of bile."

"My skin feels so greasy I have to keep taking showers. The doctors say I'm throwing off a lot of ketones."

"I did three extra enemas last night, and the pain in my kidneys isn't nearly so bad today."

"Every time I breathe, I smell this really strong whiff of motor oil. They say they have to paint the walls sometimes just to get the smell out of the rooms."

A bluff, relentlessly positive-thinking shoe salesman with lung cancer; a young English woman with cancer of the uterus, soft spoken, determined to live for the sake of her new baby; a terribly frail, once beautiful, middle-aged schoolteacher, attended by her infinitely patient husband, her stomach cancer arrested, the tumor apparently neither shrinking nor spreading; the middle-aged multiple sclerosis patient, her legs tingling, numb, so that walking was becoming a struggle—we all listened with rapt, intense hope to each other's stories of toxins released and evacuated, of former patients restored to health resuming their lives, free of the ominous, chaotic fears that had driven us here, us, "the incurables"—or so we'd been labeled by conventional medicine that, for all its ingenuity, had reached its limit in helping us. In an ironic swipe at the medical establishment, which was naturally hostile to the clinic's methods, and with not so subtle hucksterism, the clinic used that label of "incurable" in its promotional literature, attempting a little mythmaking of its own: "Incurable" could be changed into its opposite; from cranks and outcasts obsessed with our own bodily excretions, we now became the elect, the superheroes of death and disease!

We had our stars of recovery, stars more luminous in our quietly desperate eyes than Gloria Swanson or Dorothy Lamour: the Alabama housewife with a brain tumor who was given a few weeks but now, completely recovered, had written a book about her cure; or the truck farmer with an almost certainly fatal, wildfire variety of melanoma, who was now so healthy that he allowed himself a drink and cigar from time to time. An entire book chronicling the miraculous cures of the incurables was always ready at hand—we looked to it for encouragement, we convinced ourselves that our cases weren't nearly so dire, that all we needed to do to be saved was follow the regimen. And undoubtedly many were saved—the treatment did work, we met the survivors, talked with them, relived their medical histories from the abandonment by their regular doctors to their resurrection at the clinic. And of course many died— their condition was too advanced; for some physiological reason they couldn't tolerate the treatment, their immune systems were far too impaired by radiation, by chemotherapy, by sheer exhaustion.

After a few days at the clinic, as the doctors had promised, I began to have a "healing reaction." The day was hot; in the fields surrounding the clinic the weeds burned gold. Across the road from the clinic I was taking a walk in the tiny village where most of the nursing staff lived: a slab of concrete for a basketball court, small cinder-block houses painted pastel blues and with corrugated roofs, roosters and hens, dirt roads wandering up the hillside the village was on. The eerie sense of normal life going on beyond the confines of the clinic made me realize just how extreme my state of mind was—hope that I would get well, and that I could be as stolid in my health as the roosters and hens obliviously pecking at the dirt, had narrowed my attention to an obsessive concentration on my body's functioning. The drifting noise of conversation, of the sound of sweeping, of clothes being washed outdoors by hand on washboards and in tubs, of the backfire and drone of cars and small tractors, all these signs of daily domestic chores and routine labor argued against my own quiet monomania.

That my hope (and fear) could so limit my responses to the world showed me how sealed off I and my fellow sufferers were in our infinitely self-regarding battle with disease. The appalling self-involvement and secret egotism of the dying! Our tyrannical self-awareness tracked moment to moment the subtlest fluctuations in our breathing, body temperature, and heart rates, while the day-to-day world we wanted so desperately to get back to, the world of easy sleep, of unregulated food and drink, of routine contact with one another, we automatically blocked out. Oblivious to life outside the clinic, all we could think of were the mortal chances of our own sorry, aching flesh. To break ourselves of the fear of death, to face it with the apparent confidence of Socrates!

At Epidaurus, the temple of Asclepius was filled with votive offerings—marble eyes, ears, legs, hands, feet, all the parts of the body that the god had healed left behind in simulacra as a remembrance of the god's grace: the wounded arm exchanged for the well arm, the blind eye left behind for the sighted one. Long lists of cases inscribed in the stone slabs record the method of consulting the god as well as the manner of his cures. The god's way of treating wounds (dressings and cautery) and broken bones (various kinds of splints) must have seemed to the patients more common sense than miracle. But the cures that depended on supernatural intervention—the miraculous mending overnight of a broken vase, for example— tease my imagination the most; why shouldn't I wake up some morning with all my cracks seamlessly mended? But my skepticism returns; I shrug off such hopes. My oscillations between belief and doubt mirror exactly what the god's patients must have felt: it seems that in later times the efficacy of the old faith healing fell into disrepute, and the priests substituted it for elaborate prescriptions concerning diet, baths, and regimen: in many particulars quite similar to the treatment I was following in Mexico.

But here in the village, removed from the clinic, in the hot sunshine, I was outside of my obsession; my body seemed for a moment like any other body. Someone looking at me wouldn't have known from my appearance that I was sick. Why didn't I behave like Socrates in the face of my own death? To buy a rooster from a villager, slit its throat, and offer it up to Asclepius was no more eccentric than enemas, "healing reactions," and the company of other incurables. Hope? Was this alien state of mind part of the punishing operations of hope? Malignant hope that kept me frantically pursuing health? Would it be a form of suicide to refuse to compromise with mortality? To abandon hope, to inure myself to physical suffering and eventual death . . . if only I could keep my head clear of my body's special pleading, "Do this and this; you'll recover, you'll get well."

Perhaps I was addled by the heat, and certainly I was in the throes of the "healing" fever that the doctors in the clinic had predicted. But at that moment, in a village whose name I can't even remember, I felt free of the clinic! The houses' pitted cinder blocks and mortar scalloped between the courses; the wooden fences around dirt yards; the scrounged camper shells ingeniously propped on cement foundation walls and used as tool sheds and bedrooms—these imparted a sense of almost supernatural order and normalcy, of an unimpeachable certainty of well-being.

This state of well-being was impersonal: it had nothing to do with me or the relative state of my health; a diamond absolute, it held sway no matter what kind of doctor or medicine I put my trust in, no matter who got well or who died, no matter what hope promised or failed to deliver. If the clinic in its extremity mirrored the sacred groves of Asclepius—last refuge of the sick and dying—then the village that afternoon was like workaday Epidaurus, setting of unselfconscious well-being, normalcy, and order. Yet how foreign those words sound in the ears of the "incurable," inspiring both awe and despair. Though I could sense that power as operative in others' lives, I myself had never felt so far from health, even at the very moment when the sunshine and heat seemed most resplendent with health-giving qualities.

Now, when I think of Asclepius's power, I see kings as well as peasants, each praying to be healed, lying down for the night on the cold marble. I see the god in his benevolence appearing to the sleepers, filling this head and that with its own special miraculous dream. Even Alexander the Great's father, Philip of Macedon, visited Asclepius's sacred groves and left his breastplate and spear on the god's altar. But then I imagine the sick and dying whose dreams weren't colored by the god—wouldn't the god's decision to heal some but not others also make him a figure of dread? But small matter if the god favored Philip, or chose instead to cure the poorest bondsman in his kingdom: both visits would be punctiliously added to the other inscriptions, more evidence of the god's influence and power.

Shortly afterward my fever spikes, and my stay at the clinic comes to an abrupt end. My nausea and chills, my red blood cells breaking down so quickly that my urine turns black—it's quite clear to everyone that unless I get to a hospital immediately, a real hospital, I might die.

While my mother drives me toward the border and a hospital in California, I focus on the emergency as if it's someone else's body, someone else's life at stake. My mind is weirdly cool and distant, my body aches, aches and shivers; fever blurs my vision: I feel afloat in a plunging elevator, only the elevator is my body descending farther and farther from the untroubled, expanding light that is my own awareness watching, detached, invulnerably serene, unmoved by the tense voices talking far below . . . my voice, my mother's voice discussing what to say to the doctors, deciding, *No,* we can't tell them about the clinic, and, *Yes,* the body in trouble may need a blood transfusion.

The farther my body falls, the more attuned grows my perception of how weak my arms and legs feel, how light my pulse—my breathing, too, is beginning to plunge, my body and breath separate so completely that body seems infinitely heavy, stone-stupid, elemental . . . Now we've reached the emergency room, the neon keeps twisting and writhing, wrenching itself away from the fixture, then starkly dissolving into the shadows. In the bed next to mine someone is moaning about his headache, a headache so terrible that his moans create a disturbance like a heat wave, pulsating, a force field of blank pain.

From far outside my body I feel my heart speed up, beating so quickly that the darkness the neon dissolves into rises into my eyes and flows over and around me, reaching even to the place where now I'm nothing but hovering Being above my own voice crying, "I can't breathe; I don't believe I can breathe." A hand grips mine—the headache, the moans, they belong to this hand. Tears come to my eyes when I realize that no matter how fierce the pain the headache and moans spring from, the hand that belongs to this pain has come to comfort me, to calm me so that I can breathe until the nurse gets there with oxygen.

My body is still free-falling; my heart flutters so quickly and faintly it seems about to stop. I sense panic trying to pierce the spreading blackness that holds me until I hear inside my head a voice so authoritative, so utterly self-convinced and godlike that it might as well be Socrates arguing over the soul, or Asclepius come to me in a dream: "Wonder Bread builds strong bodies twelve ways, Wonder Bread builds strong bodies twelve ways, Wonder Bread . . ." The oxygen mask fits over my face, and through my strengthening breath, my brain and body begin to fuse back together; now my heart starts to slow, and the slogan from the old TV commercial, which has surfaced from my childhood, and which I used to chant to myself whenever I was worried or afraid, inscribes itself on pure untextured mind—which again feels the impress of my identity . . . and with that comes fear, naked, raw fear.

That I knew this could happen, that fever almost always results in my red blood cells' obliteration, drives home that I am ill, chronically ill, that my disease can kill me, has almost killed me. My desire to get well, my hope to return to the unconscious ease of assumed health, now seems wildly absurd. I can't stifle the voice needling in on every side, *How can you lead your life if life means that you must be ill?*

More than a decade later, I'm sitting at my mother's dining room table, still one of the incurables. I'm about to play a role that I've played many times—the survivor, "the old-timer" of death, the *philosophe* of disease. I always feel a little fraudulent—but my feelings aren't the point: my mother has invited over her neighbor's seventeen-year-old son who has lymphoma. He's tall, with an athlete's torso and legs—but his muscle tone is beginning to slacken in his chest and abs, the result of his illness's onslaught, of radiation and chemotherapy.

"I'm out of school for a while," he says, "but hey, that's okay—," and gives an ironic smile. I recognize the style of humor: slightly deadpan, rueful, making much of negatives, already he's realized that the world can't easily tolerate more direct displays of emotion.

"I'll bet it really hurts to have to miss school, huh?"

"Oh yeah, I wake up weeping every morning!"

We trade jokes back and forth, each of us instinctively understanding the fear that drives our joking, but also enjoying our shared sense of being different from other people, of being members of a club that in theory everyone belongs to, but that only some of us, and only at certain moments of our lives, are truly enrolled in.

"It's not going so bad—my hair fell out in patches so I just shaved my head. I like wearing a cap anyway, so what's the difference?"

"Hey, my hair just falls out on its own!"

Around and around we go, slipping in bits of our medical histories. The more I learn about his condition, the more despairing I feel about his chances; one reason he's asked to meet me is to let me know, a stranger uninvested in his life, what no one else near him can bear to hear: that the odds aren't good, that in a year or two he may well be dead. But it's not only despair we feel underneath the joking—our laughter is genuine: I sense in him an intense pride in carrying himself bravely, in his refusal to say too much, in his stoical restraint.

I've played this scene before in more fraught circumstances. I'll meet with a friend of a friend of a friend who's scared, vulnerable, valiantly keeping in check anxiety and dread. We talk about alternative treatments, both of us knowing that if the doctors pronounce you terminal, a miracle is required . . . and miracles, our glances agree, are in short supply . . . After these conversations I always feel drained, I wonder why I put myself in these situations: Am I kind of a death junkie, getting off on intense emotion? Does it reassure me to see someone sicker than myself?

This kind of self-accusation becomes its own dodge: how much easier for me to cocoon myself away from such people, to keep myself insulated from their pain and dread. My motives for meeting him may be less than altruistic, but wouldn't it be worse to refuse to meet this young man, so dignified in his fear, so intently matter-of-fact about the prospect of his own death? Yet in my role as elder statesman how dislocated I feel, the incurable still secretly lusting after a cure, my acceptance of my fate a not-so-subtle ruse to trick myself into thinking that my condition is as routine as the sunrise. The constant threat of mortality has shaped me the way wind shapes a tree, bending the trunk in the direction that it habitually blows. Or sometimes I think of myself as moving in a different gravitational field, the heaviness and clumsiness of my movements contrived to look almost normal. It's only when I meet up with someone like this young man that I understand the extent of my own psychic accommodation to this field's warping force. Off kilter from the sudden, strange intimacy we share, I realize I'm a little afraid of him—no, not of him but of everything he's suffered and may still suffer. Does he feel the same about me, as if fear and despair were infectious? Yet what greater consolation can we offer than the physical reassurance of our failing but still bravely persisting bodies?

I suppose the point is to overcome what is negative in these feelings, to recognize in our jokes our shared sense of a common fate, even in our veiled, perhaps mutual fear, a genuine bond. But aren't these things also sources of estrangement—from ourselves, from other people, from the world?

Now we finish talking; we say good-bye. The tension I've felt the whole time we've been together tightens inside me, I feel helpless to protect him or myself, inadequate to the enormity of the trial that each of us one day will face. I consider what may be his fate—and realize, almost with a kind of envy, that he could soon know more than I what it means to be "incurable." As I watch him walk away, unexpectedly he turns and calls out to me, "Good luck!" For a moment I'm a little ashamed; shouldn't I be the one wishing him luck, I the old-timer, "the incurable"? What have I given him, after all? Is it simply the fact that I'm still alive, striving to lead a relatively normal life, which makes me seem special in his eyes and so spurred him to seek me out? As if by pretending to be healthy in the eyes of the sick, I might slip out from under the watchful gaze of my own fate and actually cross back over the border between disease and health? Yet I, too, wanted to meet him, to share this intimacy of our estrangement from the world of free and easy flesh. How young he is, how vital his body seems despite the alien pallor beneath his tan—my hand moments ago held his, and I can still feel his skin's warmth fading from my skin.

The voice you dream is mine—bend down to me, come listen; I'm one of Asclepius's yellow snakes, the one his hand reaches out to; or else I'm his dog stretched dozing under his chair. In snake language, in dog language, he whispers why you people suffer, why you, among all these others, are fated to get well, and why you, with the same illness, already belong to the gods of the underworld. His voice in my head inhabits the marble of his statue, the stone so cool against me reassuring in its chill. You patients who leave me offerings, I barely notice you, I'm so intent on the delicious cool that rises and flows through me . . . As I lie here, my belly listens to the marble, I hear it whispering to me in the voice of the god. At night when you're asleep and my tongue licks your ear, you too may learn what the god knows. Bend down to me, come listen, in the god's own words, to the reason for your life and death, the reason for your suffering and pain, the reason why the god will or will not heal you.

brendan wolfe

Here is a brief and personalized profile of a symphony, what it means and what it might have meant to one young musician—combined with a disillusioning moment that redirected his life.

this is not a review
of shostakovich's
fifth symphony

Instead, it is me trying to remember the beginning, sitting here with the lights turned low and the clicking hum of my ceiling fan, trying to remember. For Dr. Culver it had been like quoting Shakespeare or the Bible. Standing in the carpeted lobby at Symphony Hall in Chicago, we asked him something about the Shostakovich cello concerto. "Oh sure!" he exclaimed and vigorously hummed the opening bars in perfect tune. Even under such a shower of saliva we were dumbstruck. After that we tried to stump him, with names like Hindemith and Piston, but it never worked. It was as if a full symphony orchestra had taken up residence in his head, on a moment's call. I, on the other hand, am forced to settle for the compact disc. The New York Philharmonic, Leonard Bernstein conducting, recorded live at Bunka Kaikan, Tokyo, 1979. I press PLAY and I can hear it now; I can finally remember now. It begins as good symphonies do, quietly, and as all Shostakovich symphonies do, darkly. Moderato. D Minor. It begins with an anapest, or nearly an anapest—one short, then long—referring to Beethoven's Fifth. And there is a low conversation among the strings: first the cellos, then the violins, in hushed tones. They are huddled in the back shadows, whispering over shoulders, periodically working themselves to a nervous pitch; the violins suddenly screaming—then just as suddenly cut off. The temperatures here are subzero, we are shivering, and there are these silences everywhere. Held breaths. Pianissimo. These are the moments most difficult for musicians to master because they are where the fear inhabits. The fear that causes us to play and to listen and to write and to read in the first place. And it is inside of these silences that I am able to sit once again on the cold tile of a second-floor classroom turned dressing room. It is Variety Show, my sophomore year in high school. I am dressed in a wretched black polyester tuxedo and next to me is Heather listening to her headphones again. She also plays violin and has bright, curly red hair. She looks a bit like a Raggedy Ann doll. I suspect that she is a smoker, partly because her dad is an artist. They sometimes give me rides home from Youth Symphony on Saturdays, driving across town in congested traffic, listening to the radio. They were surprised when I had not even heard of a group like R.E.M., and I can't help it if I don't understand why her father, even if he does paint, knows about music. This makes no sense to me. Now she asks me to put on the headphones because she has recorded this Shostakovich symphony from the radio. "Who is Shostakovich?" I ask, and she tells me that they played Symphony no. 5 in Youth Symphony last year, except that I hadn't been in Youth Symphony last year. I listen and at first I hate it. I feel like I am listening to a skeleton. The bass tiptoes across the score while the woodwinds very carefully repeat back the theme, note for note. There is no room for error here, comrades. It is so quiet I can hear the audience shifting in their seats. I borrow the tape from Heather, take it home to my room in the basement, and listen to it again and again, playing it loudly, as if it were rock music. I do not understand that this is something Heather and I now share. Perhaps if I do I should fall in love with her as she has fallen in love with me, always referring to me in those melodramatic notes we pass as "dear friend." After all, Shostakovich is no small thing to have in common. Many years later I would check out his memoir from the library and look at pictures of him. Dmitry Dmitryevich. He was small, wiry, with round, black-rimmed glasses, thin, bloodless lips, and streaks of black hair pasted across his head. He wrote about receiving two scathing reviews in *Pravda* in 1936—reviews he attributed to Comrade Stalin himself—and the terrible, throat-catching fear that he had endured. The subjects of such reviews routinely disappeared. But he did not, an even more terrible fate, he surmised, for it only doubled, or maybe tripled, his fearfulness. This is how it was in Soviet Russia, he wrote. But in 1937 he triumphed with his Fifth Symphony. A Soviet artist's reply to just criticism, it has been said. Others have called it a complete capitulation. After the great pessimism of the first movement, the finale rejoices. "The rejoicing is forced," Shostakovich wrote in his memoir, "created under threat, as in *Boris Godunov*. It's as if someone were beating you with a stick and saying, 'Your business is rejoicing, your business is rejoicing' . . ." For this reason, some see Shostakovich as a *yurodivy,* a "holy fool," a jester. He is mocking us with this symphony. The audience at its premier is said to have wept. And I do not care about his finale, anyway. I'm playing my tape so loudly my mom is forced to ask me to turn it down (against her better judgment, it would seem, "because at least the boy is listening to something decent down there"), but I hear only the Moderato, the first movement. I hear its emptiness and its doubts. It is so melancholy, but not in a wistful way, not in a nostalgic way; rather, it is irascible, delusional, and manic depressive, characterized by furious outbursts from the brass sections followed abruptly by soothing chords from the violins. For me, it is lonely and full of omens. It is full of who I felt I was in high school. I did not learn to love Symphony no. 5 or even understand it on a technical level. I press PLAY and I am listening to my mirror. I am sitting in the poorly lit high school cafeteria late one evening after school, where we are practicing our string quartet. We are struggling with the Allegro finale of Shostakovich's String Quartet no. 1 in C. This time I am playing viola ("only different from a violin," Dr. Culver says, "because it burns longer"); in fact, this is the first piece I have ever played on viola. It is frantic and utterly overwhelming, but we are assured that it is "a little Symphony no. 5," written just one year later, in 1938, and this is why we agree to learn it. I have trouble concentrating, though, because I am desperately in love with Michele, the first violin, and I know that she doesn't love me, but instead a boy she affectionately calls "shithead." (Wagnerian tragedy, this. I am turned black inside, so that Heather writes me a note saying that I am letting my feelings "slowly destroy" me.) And I can't stop thinking about how this scene is so perfect: the four of us in the shadowy, abandoned cafeteria, our music echoing off the walls and plastic chairs. This is something I should write about, a *danse macabre,* describing the notes leaping off the pages and sliding down the stands. They fence in the salad bar, joust by the pop machine, and kiss under the skylight, before roving off to commit unthinkable acts of double-deed. My story unravels in rapturous and sinister fashion, plagued with doubt and unbearable emotion. I want to net Shostakovich with my words; I desperately want to decode and communicate the many colors, textures, and timbres his music realizes inside of me. Of course, such stories remain unwritten because I am too afraid to fail, because failure is inevitable, and I cannot bear it after failing on my instruments, failing to live up to my desires. This is the incidental music of my life. Several years later the four of us are together again, this time playing a wedding reception in a Knights of Columbus banquet hall. We wait until everyone is good and drunk and then we pull out String Quartet no. 1. We shock them, just like we wanted to, and amuse them, because this is our incidental music and not theirs. When I do finally ask Michele to the prom—we're on the phone and I have the script of my question written out in front of me—she answers she's not sure if she'll be in town that weekend but she'll let me know. She'll call me. And already I can hear the timpani roll of betrayal. I later learn she played Shostakovich that night, a quartet gig I turned down. Now I wish that this is something that Michele and I do not share, I want to turn back the clock on Shostakovich, because how can she understand what it means to me? The violins are increasingly insistent with the second theme; they strike their octaves impatiently, until finally they settle down into a peaceful, almost beautiful, interlude. But a wind picks up, first in the violas, then the flute, punctuated by a pounding piano, swirling through the orchestra, picked up by the brass, and the martial announcements of the snare, a screaming crescendo. Fortissimo. And then it is gone. It is cold and it is quiet. I am sweating and shivering. This is my first semester at college and I have not played my viola since the previous spring when we performed Vivaldi's Requiem for a church gig. One of my string pegs had broken—swelled up in the heat and humidity, then snapped in two. The string remained tightly wound, though, and during the performance I was forced to adjust the intonation with a pair of pliers we had retrieved from Michele's truck. Now only recently has it been repaired and I am standing unsteadily in a tiny cubicle somewhere inside the music building. This year, for its first concert, the university orchestra shall perform Shostakovich's Symphony no. 5 in D Minor, op. 47, and I intend to be a part of it. Before me sit James Dixon, legendary conductor and friend of Leonard Bernstein, and William Preucil, director of violas. I begin to play my Schubert and am almost immediately cut off by a simple wave of Dixon's hand. The verdict back so soon? "Brevity," Dr. Culver, bearded and sage, so oft announced, "is the handmaiden of concision." I bring my viola down from my chin and my hands sweat so that I think I might drop it. "What, Mr. Wolfe, did you say your major was?" Dixon asks. Clearing my throat: "English." "Yes, yes, yes . . . We do have plenty of viola majors this year, do we not, Mr. Preucil?" In this rather unremarkable way, my career as a musician ends. The fortissimo has disappeared. The strings are muted now, *con sordino,* and we have found our interlude again. The violas and cellos are all the heartbeat we have, barely pulsing, while the flute solos, then the piccolo, the oboe, then the clarinet, the violas, and the cellos are barely pulsing. There is not any more shivering, the air is too icy, and out of the highest register sounds the solo violin, with only the smallest touch of vibrato, fading on a high F. The last three and a half beats of the first movement are silent. And the music is marked *morendo.*

john t. price

"Night Rhythms" captures a dramatic sequence of events, but the power of the narrator makes the essay riveting. John T. Price writes with a pressured and unrelenting intensity. Using hard-edged and precise detail, he can be lyrical and poetic. The essay takes an interesting and decisive turn when Dr. Van Skeldt becomes a driving force in the story—and the key to the magic and healing moment that helps tie all of the characters together.

night rhythms

I leave Dean's bedside to make 2 A.M. rounds. His are the only lights, besides those in the nursing station, that are on. The inpatient unit at the children's hospital is dim and empty—silent except for a metallic hum that can be heard, just barely, in the air. I am in my nursing assistant uniform, white, except for the splotch of creamed ham I spilled on the leg during a now distant daytime meal. Besides Dean, there are ten other patients, all children, the oldest nineteen, only three years younger than I. They are all disabled—cerebral palsy, spina bifida, failure-to-thrive, hyperactivity. But that is during the day. They are asleep now, free from their daytime gnawings and spasms.

My job tonight is to go from one room to the next, checking diapers and catheters. There are not many to check this round. So I just listen to their breathing, and if it is too silent, I place my hand on their rib cages, gently, to feel the measure of their sleep. I am glad it is not the designated hour to reposition them, to wake them up, interrupt, and, if they have had surgery, to cause them pain. That time is two hours away. For now, I can just watch and feel for their breath, celebrating the trail of drool for what it means: peace. Sleep the elixir. I am extra quiet.

I return to Dean's bedside once again, alone. There is a blue swelling near his ankle where, earlier in the evening, Dr. Van Skeldt tried to insert an IV needle, again and again. It was clear then that we would have to transfer him to the main hospital, where they are better equipped to deal with him. Dr. Van Skeldt has left to make arrangements. The night nurse enters, her support hose rubbing and swishing, to register what vitals she can. "Why did he bring him here in the first place?" she says. "He knew we wouldn't be able to take care of him. He knew that." But the care facility won't take him back, I remind her. Maybe this is the only place he has. "Well, I don't know about that."

She is right in a way; our small unit isn't equipped to handle a patient like Dean. But nevertheless he is lying in a bed here. Dean won't live much longer. He has severe cerebral palsy, which means he choked during birth, which means the rhythm of the contractions was wrong. His lungs opened too soon. He has lived seventeen years, barely. I have been with Dean tonight for over two hours, just sitting on the side of his bed and watching his rib cage extend then collapse: up . . . down . . . up, up, up . . . down. His lips, dry, are collecting a thin film of mucus. His auburn hair shines with nearly three days' oil. He is so emaciated that when the fluorescent light casts blue upon his twisted limbs, it sends shadows in odd places, unexpected: pelvis, upper lip, ribs . . .

An hour later I leave to clean the sunroom. This is the children's playroom, now empty. Around me the carpet, the plastic chairs and tables are covered with the daytime patterns of childhood, lingering. Toys and pieces of toys lay here and there, always everywhere, weaving together messy spirals and rhythms and textures. Yellow, red, blue. Minihouses, Ken heads, Fisher-Price farms, hollow plastic bulbs—some together, some not. I pick them up, one by one, and put them in their designated places. I used to work the evening shift here, just after supper, when the sunroom is full of children, of wet hair and pajamas; movement and noise; tricycles, storybooks, gossip; house, cops, robbers; tossing, chasing, shouting. John, John, John, they called from all corners, all sides. The supervisor's big butt, Dan's booger, Kara's farts. Faster and faster, the kinetic energy of their play seemed to raise the small hairs on my neck and arms . . . But I'd forget. On the mat, near the television, would be the other patients like Dean. Quiet, except for tiny rockings from seizures or masturbation. Movement would flurry about them, balls would accidentally bounce off their heads as we nursing assistants played with the other children; all of us believing, hoping, that because these patients lay quietly, just breathing and rocking, they were pacified. With bright colors spinning around us, we would tuck them and their gnarled fingers into the backs of our minds and forget them. But here on the night shift I remember.

I return to Dean's bedside. His steamer is stuttering. I lift off the top and add another pint of distilled water. James, my only brother, is on my mind tonight. He was buried fifteen years ago in soft blue, terry-cloth pajamas at a funeral I wasn't allowed to attend. A stillborn, lost during labor. I sometimes dream about that funeral, but not very often anymore. In fact, I haven't thought of James much at all recently. But tonight is different. From Dean's windows I can see a distant intersection, where the traffic lights are changing by themselves. Green, yellow, red, again and again . . . no one is awake to heed them except me. I am on the night shift, and I feel as if I am privy to the secrets of day existence; privy to the secret knowledge that pedestrian buttons on traffic lights are an illusion. There is no real control. The traffic lights change according to timers, predetermined rhythms that go unnoticed during the day like the regular seizures of children who lay on playroom mats. But at night I can see them changing while others sleep.

It seems unimportant, unless you realize that just over the curve of the earth, surrounding our sleeptime, are daytime lands and cities where people and machines are pounding and cars jam clover-leaf junctions and planes are landing and emerging through thunder. People barbecuing, starving, mowing lawns, riding camels or tugboats or the backs of lovers in pounding, ceaseless, pulsating patterns and rhythms that blend into palimpsestic nonsense until just once—just once—the synchronization goes bad, and you find yourself standing near a Dean and counting the number of times his rib cage rises, watching as a doctor jabs and jabs and jabs an IV needle into the tender flesh of his foot in the hope of finding a vessel with a pulse. Or you find yourself a woman in labor, in an empty hospital room in April, whimpering as you feel the frantic kicking against your abdomen slowly dwindle to silence. Or you find yourself a father standing outside your remaining son's doorway, the night before Easter, letting the heavy candy drop from your hand and onto the carpet, one by one by one. Or, at seven, you find yourself alone, tearing out your hair in fists because secretly, for some forgotten reason, you had once wished the baby dead, and indeed it had been born so.

Dean coughs, just a little, then returns to the wet labor of his breathing. Softly, carefully, I slip my thumb into his small velvet palm and caress the top of his hand with my index finger. I don't know if he notices, but I feel the need. The need to shout him on, to set the pace of his life stream, to fill arteries and lungs and heart with the measure of strong, rosy-cheeked life. On my caress he'll live out the evening, keep breathing, stop choking, become born. Or so I imagine. But who is this boy to me, anyway? Why am I drawn to him? Perhaps because James was my brother, and because I was the only male child, out of three, to survive birth. Perhaps because James was born at night, and because it was a night nurse who left my mother in a room alone. Perhaps Dean is what James would have been if he had lived, a good portion of his brain suffocated. Perhaps I am just unusually sensitive tonight. I don't know. I don't know why I'm sitting here. Why, out of the hundreds of children I've assisted in this place, some terminally ill, I should feel the need to especially comfort this boy on this night. I just do. So I sit and I caress and I listen, beneath the hum of machines, for the breath of life, and the secret rhythms of compassion.

. . .

Too quickly, Dr. Van Skeldt enters the room, and the night nurse is with him. They have brought a cart for the transfer. He has decided not to use motor transport, and I wonder why. Why push him when you could drive him the short, bumpy distance to Main? I don't know a lot about Dr. Van Skeldt except that he arrived from Boston, is divorced, and lives alone, no children. Usually, he walks around the halls with a grave brow, checking a file or a patient or two, rarely going too far out of his way for patient or staff. He's considered rather cold.

But his relationship to Dean has been an enigma for everyone. Among staff, Dean is referred to as Dr. Van Skeldt's personal "project." He checks in on Dean every evening, meeting with staff in the process, courteously begging favors from us for his care: Could you put a pillow there please? And tonight, when Dean whimpered as the needle kept missing its mark, I thought I read, on Dr. Van Skeldt's brow, a wrinkle of pain. He has had to move Dean from one facility to the next, trying to find a place willing to take care of him until he dies. Now we can't keep him either.

Dr. Van Skeldt takes the two far ends of Dean's bed sheet, and I grab the near. Slowly we lift him, with the nurse's help, from his bed to the cart. Dean's eyes are moving back and forth, and his breath stretches to squeak out a whimper. He is crying, I can tell, and frightened. Slowly we start to move—Dr. Van Skeldt in front, me in back—past the nurse, out the door and onto the cracked sidewalk that leads to the main hospital. It is an Iowa summer at night. It is a time when the slopes and lulls of the river valley bear the thick steam of vegetable life, soaking the fur of rabbits as they nibble, calling witness to the indisputable fact that the earth itself breathes. In the air is the smell of damp earth, and the faint hint of late-blooming lilacs. Suddenly, we stop moving.

"Now isn't that pretty?" Dr. Van Skeldt says to himself, or maybe to Dean. "I caught that scent earlier. I was hoping it would still be here for us. It reminds me of California when I was a boy. During those summers the smell from those blossoms filled the air. My mother used to say that if you breathed too much of it you would faint away or lose your socks or something. That's what she used to say then. There it is again . . . isn't that something?"

Dr. Van Skeldt pauses, then touches Dean's shoulder, lightly. He checks the IV pole. And then we move on, toward the bright fluorescent lights of Main.

barbara helen berger

There are many cathartic and illuminating moments in this touching and unusual essay—from recognizing the literal beauty of a bone to acknowledging the longing that comes prior to the burst of creativity in art or writing or science and connecting creativity to the makeup of the human body. The metaphor of bone is ever enduring—from her father's bone cancer to the dead bones in the box to the bones scattered in her father's final resting place in the sea.

bones

We were the only kids in the neighborhood with a real human skeleton in our house. Every year on Halloween, Dad carried it up from the basement to stand by the front door, just inside. We'd run home from school to put on our gypsy bangles and pirate capes, and the skeleton would be there. "Mr. Bones!"

There were plenty of hats to dress up in, but Mr. Bones could never wear one. A stainless steel hook, by which he hung from the skeleton stand, came up through the bare skull. So instead of a hat, Dad tied a red bandanna around the neck, over the shoulder blades in back, the clavicles in front. It looked quite casual. Then he inserted the stem of a white chrysanthemum between Mr. Bones's teeth.

The rest of the year, Mr. Bones stayed in the basement, next to the roaring furnace. He belonged to that world down there in the rooms where Dad worked, with microscopes and the cameras with black accordion bellows, film hanging from clotheslines, drawing tables piled with papers, brushes, pens, and over the windows, shelves filled with specimens in jars.

Up in my room at night, it was not Mr. Bones who haunted me. It was the fetus I saw one time, white as milk, floating in one of those jars. Through a thin amniotic veil, I saw tiny human fingers and eyes like small black beads.

Most of the jars held things only Dad could name, tissues turned in on themselves or stretched and pinned like a patch of cloth. In one big crock was a stomach, wrinkled and pale as an antique silk from Great-Grandmother's attic trunk. When Dad wasn't home, we charged a nickel to let the neighbor kids see the stomach. They peered into the shadows, too, where the skeleton stood. Then we ran back upstairs.

Mr. Bones was always there, though he might be in pieces. Dad often took him apart. With a fine saw he cut through the skull, leaving the cranial dome intact. Then he cut down through the nose and jaw and opened the face like a book. He could read the intricate hollows inside. He knew them from years of medical school and years bent over in surgery—cutting, clamping, and stitching. But he loved drawing and painting even more.

This was our bond, Dad's and mine. I loved drawing and painting, too. I'd come downstairs and stand by the slanted desk, watching him work while a cigarette burned in the ashtray and Glen Miller tunes played on his radio. With the model of bones beside him, he'd make a careful drawing. Then he would paint not only the bones but all the soft tissues, in layers of shaded color. He'd dip a fine brush in white tempera, dab it just so, and the painted tissues looked moist, translucent, shining. He made the horror of an open skull with all the mysteries inside it a thing of beauty.

When he was done, Dad put the bones together again with wire and wing nuts on slender bolts. If you asked, he'd tell you the name of any bone in the skeleton and how it fit with the rest. He'd tell you how everything grew in the embryo when cells became brain and blood and beating heart. He let you in on the marvels, the treasures of his own amazement. The more he learned and the more he knew, he said, the more he saw the order of the universe, alive in every detail of the body. My dad loved this order, the vast intelligence behind it. He didn't call it God, a name too badly scarred by brimstone and fire shot from the pulpits of his childhood. But the way he spoke, I knew what my dad saw in the bones was holy.

Then one summer, home from my first year at college, I saw it, too, for myself. All year in the art school, I had been drawing. I didn't want to stop. One hot day, I took my big pad of paper and drawing pencils down into the coolness of Dad's workroom.

"Dad, can I borrow a bone?"

"Sure, sweetie," he said. He gave me a tibia, I think it was. One of the long leg bones.

My hand had learned to follow my eye while my eye followed the contours of things, as if to touch by seeing. So with hand and eye and the point of a 6B pencil, I searched out the contour of that bone on the empty white paper. It was the only bone in the world. I explored the full length of its shape, discovering subtle curves and ridges. Then all at once, I saw its sheer grace.

This was more than sculpture. Every nuance of form in the bone had grown just so for a purpose, for the root of a muscle, the motion of a joint, the life of a living whole. Dad might have handed me any bone in the skeleton—a rib, a vertebra—any one of them would have shown me its own particular grace. And then, to think of each bone finding its shape from the few cells in every embryo that grow into a human being, a bird, a dog, a horse, a fish—the genius of it all was too immense. I began to cry.

Dad came to my side. "What's wrong?"

I shook my head and picked up the bone, to hold this one human tibia in my hands until I could speak.

"It's so perfect. So beautiful."

He only nodded, and laid his hand on my shoulder. The revelation was sealed for me by that warm hand, the weight of it resting there, then the gentle pat, pat and his voice saying softly, "Carry on."

I kept on drawing, and painting, through the rest of my college years and beyond. I learned there are times when no revelation happens. The pencil or brush is dead in my hand. Vision seems to be utterly lost, swallowed up in some inner darkness. Then all I have is longing. Before there is even a vague shape floating in the mind like tissue in a glass, there is only the longing. I never knew anyone, not even Dad, who could say where it comes from, or why.

He did say, "Well, we just have to create. Human beings seem to be made that way."

It helped to regard the ache of longing itself as a sign of something so basic, primordial as a seed in the earth.

"Dad," I said one day, "could I please borrow Mr. Bones? There's a painting I need to do."

"Sure," he said.

By that time, Dad was retired. No more deadlines or medical journals, he did his art for himself. Mr. Bones was retired, too, in a closet.

"Take him home to your studio. Keep him as long as you like."

So, padded with blankets, Mr. Bones came home with me in the back of my station wagon. Legs and arms rattled and swung to life when I hoisted the heavy skeleton stand and staggered into my studio. Same old bones. Same old saw cuts held together with wire, wing nuts, and bolts. Ah, here you are. My old friend. Why did we still call him Mr. Bones? He was actually a woman. Dad had even said so himself long ago, "You can tell by the pelvis." This woman was very small, from Asia he thought. Yet I never did wonder about her, who she was, her life, her death, who she'd left behind. The naked fact of her bones was always enough. Sister Bones, human bones, woman or man, she was universal.

Now she stood in the corner, a silent model. I piled a few books under the hanging feet, to approximate a standing pose, even a contrapposto. I stretched a tall canvas and primed it with sanded white. Day by day, a drawing grew on the canvas. Then a painting grew on the drawing. I dabbed and scumbled and glazed, shaded the curves and colors of bone, faintly gold like old ivory, the spaces between and around the bones a humus of deep umbers. Day by day, in layers of paint, a vine grew up between the skeleton's feet. Glowing with soft, dry-brushed light, sprouting leaves as it went, the vine wound its way up through the open spaces of pelvis and ribs, up through the whole figure of bones standing there in the earthen dark. Four buds were just beginning to bloom around the skull. After a day of work, before bed, I'd come back into the studio, to the solitude and smells of paint and whatever light filtered in from the moon. The shadowy bones on the easel were a comfort. I came simply to sit and gaze, take root in the emerging vision, lean into the axis of my life before I lay down to sleep.

You live with a painting inside and out, and it grows into a kind of mirror. It comes into being by the work of your own hands and yet this image, a new life, looks back at you with more than you know. What I see there is always more than myself.

So it was, sometime later, walking one day in the city. I thought of my own bones. In my mind's eye I saw the skull balancing on the spine, vertebrae holding me up, femurs and tibias swinging, metatarsals bearing my weight. Then I imagined the bones of those all around me, people rushing to cross the streets, striding along with briefcases and bags. Under umbrellas, jackets, and coats, we all carried our sorrows and dreams on the same slender bones. We weren't much bigger than birds in the roar between tall buildings, under the sky. Some crushing fate could fall onto any one of us. Tenderness swept over me in a wave. How strange, how strong, how fragile we are.

Even the ring of a telephone can rip the night open. Dad had a heart attack. I rushed to meet the aid car and saw his body leap into the air when they shocked his heart back to life. A few years later, they found a cancer in his throat. A surgeon cut the larynx out, and Dad's voice with it. Now he spoke with a battery-driven buzz pressed to his throat. Somehow, the true tone of him still came through. Then he lost the vision in one eye. Slowly that eye grew blank as a clouded moon. He kept it hidden most of the time behind a black lens in his glasses. Then before long the vision dimmed in his other eye. He stepped with the searching gait of an old man. Yet still he climbed up and down the stairs to his workroom, to feel his way among the familiar tools, to work at his own art.

One day the doctors found the cancer again. In his lung. In the bone of his spine.

"Well," he said, "this is it."

He wanted to die at home. So we moved a hospital bed into the living room. Mom, my sister, my brother, and I did our best to nurse him, pouring our love into any small thing, a straw to his mouth, a pillow turned, while every day he sank further into the bed. His eyes deepened into their orbits, one a dull moon, the other still bright, but he could not see even the vague shapes and shadows of us bending over the bed. He began to see something else. It was clear, he said, like the sunlit air of a spring day. "So clear, I can see every twig."

It was December, cold outside and dark. He lifted a tremulous finger to point out into the room.

"Look at that light coming in." The drapes were closed. It didn't matter. "Gold, golden light, like that painter, who is it?"

I thought . . . "Rembrandt?"

"Yes. Like Rembrandt's light. It's everywhere."

The very atoms of him must have been moving apart, leaving greater space between. He was porous to something more. Growing transparent.

"This is very interesting," he said, but he could not tell us more. There were too many tremors, too much pain, and the buzzing metal cylinder dropped from his hand.

We woke to a large stillness two mornings later. No more breath. Only a silence rising up through the house, arching over and embracing us, invisible and somehow radiant at the same time. The silence lingered around us, even while expanding out beyond the walls.

. . .

I still wait for a whisper in my inner ear, *carry on* . . . I still wish for the one warm hand to rest on my shoulder.

The only bodily presence left was in a small box from the funeral home. I imagined the roar of a furnace I never saw, the fierce alchemy that turned my dad's bones into dust. The box had weight, more than ash from a fire of wood. Every day Mom laid her hand on the box, and five years went by before it was time to give the dust back to the earth, or to the sea.

On a fine September day, we all sailed out in a boat. Mom, my aunt, my sister and brother, a few cousins, a few friends, and a man in a kilt with a bagpipe under his arm—we sailed out to raise a final toast to Dad and to scatter his ashes over Puget Sound. The tossed gray dust and bits of bone caught the sunlight as they fell. None of us expected that, the way the ashes sparkled as they sank into the green depth below. Then we scattered red and yellow dahlias, roses, daisies and watched the flowers float serenely away.

Today Sister Bones and I are alone in my studio once more. She stands in the corner, dear old friend. A large sheet of paper waits on the easel, pinned to a board. It has been there for weeks. One stroke of sunlight brushes across it, brighter than white, but leaves no mark. I have not been able to work—there is only the longing. Bouquets of pencils and brushes wait. Tubes of color wait, color in jars and color in sticks, trays of them laid out and waiting.

But now there is a whisper, a sigh in my inner ear. I don't know if it's Dad I hear or the breath of my own mind. *"Go into the marrow. Go into the marrow."*

With aching arms I lift Sister Bones down from the hook of the skeleton stand. Her bones rattle gently, hollow wooden chimes in a wind. I lay her down on the floor. Then I stretch out beside her.

We are the same size. Bone for bone we are alike, from the heels up to the pelvic brim, along the spine through the cage of ribs. Her arm touches mine. I take her finger bones in my hand. We lie here together, the floor holding us up, and below it, the earth. Clouds swim over the skylite above. Theirs is a noble pace, slow as grief.

The blue of their ocean stretches on and on completely at ease. I breathe it in. Then turn my head. Sister Bones is looking into my eyes.

Her two hollow orbits mirror my own. She sees through me, deep under the skin where vines of intricate vessels and nerves weave this life around my bones. I close my eyes. I feel my lungs empty and fill again with a deeper breath. I feel the heat of a tear leaving the corner of one eye, running down past my ear. I feel my heart beating here in the dark, faithful and soft under the breast-bone. And inside the bone, I sense a light, a core of light in all the bones, flowing like a sap with a will to bloom. There is still time. Soon, soon now I will stand up. Soon, I will begin.

tracy kidder

Tracy Kidder is a conduit—not a character—in this excerpt from *Old Friends*, relating the many dimensions of his story through the points of view of the people about whom he is writing. Kidder believes that nonfiction needn't be written in the first person to be creative; a writer can make himself known without the first person "I."

old friends

Once the theater gets in the blood, it never leaves. Eleanor was living proof at eighty. She sat in her armchair in her room on the west wing. She gazed out her window at the wintry landscape, making mental notes about the coming dress rehearsal. "I should have had a property person. Well, here's Eva's wig and Simon Legree's whip. Supposedly the piano tuner will help lower the pitch. They're all going to be terribly nervous with their families here. The lights and the PA system make *me* terribly nervous. But that's typical of the day before a performance."

Some things had gone perfectly today. Eleanor finally got, after weeks of requests, a baked Idaho potato for lunch. Her blood sugar was good at 7 A.M. and was probably better now because of the potato. On top of that, some young woman she'd never seen before, someone visiting a relative here, had given Eleanor a hat. "Oh, what a lovely beret," Eleanor said to the stranger as they were passing each other in the hall, and just like that, the young woman took off her hat and presented it to Eleanor. Not that Eleanor really cared about clothes, but she knew a fine thing when she saw it. She liked the way it looked on her in the mirror. "A beret for the bon vivant," she said. And as for the rehearsal, well, c'est la vie. Eleanor sighed toward the pine trees outside her window. "Well, if we haven't done anything else, we've created a little adrenaline in these people." She meant her fellow residents.

"Hi-*lo!*" said an extremely cheerful voice from the doorway. Eleanor's roommate, Elgie, a large smiling woman in a dress, came in, pushing the wheels of her wheelchair while padding along with her feet—the caterpillar walk.

Eleanor glanced at her. "You can come in now. I'm going."

The remark didn't seem to faze Elgie. "Well, I hope the dress rehearsal goes lovely."

"It won't," Eleanor said.

Elgie laughed heartily, a high-pitched laugh with a master-of-ceremonies quality about it.

Eleanor stiffened at the sound. "They never do," she said.

"That's what I've heard," Elgie said.

Eleanor got up, picked up her cane, her script, a bonnet, a small riding crop, and a brown wig, and headed for the door with her small quick dainty steps. Elgie's voice trailed after her, saying, "Good-bye and good luck to you. God bless you all."

Eleanor had decided to call the coming production a cabaret. In fact, it was mainly an old-fashioned minstrel show—without blackface, lest she offend racial sensitivities. Eleanor had assembled most of the materials herself, culling skits and music from the faded pages of her father's old repertoire.

One of Eleanor's most vivid childhood memories was of traveling around upstate New York early in the century, with her young mother and middle-aged impresario father, as he put on his gypsy theatrical shows. Her father would go from one small town to another, bearing large black trunks full of props. He'd recruit local talent and direct them in a minstrel show. He wrote the skits, music, and lyrics. Part of the production would take place outdoors, when he'd lead a parade of the actors down the main street, half the town strutting along behind him and most of the rest watching from the sidewalks, in those days long before television. The company would promenade to the strains of a march Eleanor's father had written, called "The Minstrel Street Parade." The chorus went like this:

Ta ta ta tum
On they come
Look at 'em mash
Hear the drums crash
Comedians in line
Some of old time
'Tis the minstrel street parade.

Her father got paid out of the receipts from the indoor per-
formances, usually staged under the auspices of the town's domi-
nant church. He always claimed it as the church of his faith,
becoming a Methodist in a Methodist town, for example, though he
was actually Episcopalian. Eleanor wrote a short book about her father—she had it published privately. "In 1915 we were still in the
north country and I performed in my first minstrel show," she
wrote. Among other acts, she sang a song called "Only a Waif."

A sad-eyed, raggedly dressed little girl of five singing "Only a
waif out in the street asking a penny from all." I would sing
my song and then walk down the aisles, supreme tragedy, as I
pretended to beg for a penny from people in the audience. Of
course, I never took any money although the patrons would
willingly have put the coins in my outstretched hands while
tears streamed down their cheeks. Although only five, I can
remember it even now, the odd satisfying sensation of making
people feel sad because of my tragic appeal.

Reminiscing about that time, back when she was allowed to be
one of the party, Eleanor said, "We trouped around the countryside,
and then I went back to being a little schoolgirl in Glens Falls." She
never got over that early experience. Deep down, she'd been restless
ever since.

Eleanor relocated to Linda Manor nearly a year ago under most
unusual circumstances. She checked herself in. What's more, she

did so without prodding from family or friends and without the compulsion of grave illness. Eleanor lived previously in a retirement home for women, a venerable Northampton institution housed in a mansion not far from Smith College. Time had worn the old building to an elegant shabbiness. Each inhabitant still had her own silver napkin ring, and a sign on the old-fashioned elevator warned against using it during electrical storms.

The retirement home was clean. Although she had to share a bathroom with several other women, Eleanor had her own cozy private bedroom. Since she'd left, many people had asked her why she'd wanted to trade that life of relative independence and privacy for confinement in a nursing home. Eleanor's answers had by now a well-rehearsed quality. Her rest-home room had become insufferably hot in the summers, she'd say. She'd recall that one day her diabetes had flared up dangerously, adding that her own mother had died that way, in a diabetic coma. Although the rest home kept a nurse on duty around the clock, Eleanor would say that she felt she needed more nursing care, or soon would. And besides, there were no men at the rest home—well, there had been one, but he didn't count—and she'd found most of her fellow female residents too prim and proper. "They're all ladies," she'd say. "They never wear pants. They never say anything risqué." But then again, people who had known Eleanor over the years said that she always came up with good reasons for making a change in her life or for leaving a place.

Eleanor's son wasn't surprised when she called him to say that she was leaving the rest home for Linda Manor. He figured she'd exhausted the rest home's theatrical possibilities, both the figurative and literal ones. In fact, Eleanor had already put on seven plays at the rest home and had begun to find the resources for casting there much too limited. "There were only ten people I could work with." She visited Linda Manor, on a social call, the summer after it opened and liked the looks of the place. "There's so much I could do here," she said.

Relatives almost always assume the considerable burden of

managing a move such as Eleanor's. But her two daughters lived far away, and, Eleanor insisted, she preferred not to trouble her son, who lived in Pittsfield. She also allowed that she had never been a very "family-oriented" person, adding that theater people rarely are. She made her decision to move and then asked for her children's approval.

Eleanor didn't have much money. She had to enroll in Medicaid. The regulations said that if she did not prepay her funeral expenses, the state would take the money. So Eleanor was obliged to prepare her own funeral shortly after she arrived at Linda Manor. The mortician called on her there. It took three hours to get everything picked out, the newspapers in which she wanted her obituary to appear, the accoutrements of the ceremony, the urn for her ashes. Every day for three weeks afterward, she felt like weeping. "And I'm not a weeper," she said, adding, of her funeral, "I think I'm more afraid of going through with it now that I've paid for it." She would like five more years. And in five more years, she figured, she would wish for another five.

Linda Manor wasn't all that Eleanor had hoped. She disliked the food generally and detested her roommate Elgie. She often spoke yearningly of the three private rooms, each occupied by a person paying the private rate. She'd never be able to pay for one of those rooms herself, but, Eleanor reasoned, she was doing a great deal for the nursing home in the way of arranging and managing activities for residents. She felt herself really to be more like one of the staff than a resident. So perhaps some arrangement could be made when one of the private rooms' occupants expired. Any of them might go at any time, Eleanor thought. Meanwhile, she was keeping busy. Speaking about one of the women in the room next door to hers, Eleanor said, "She has *no* memory, and she doesn't have Alzheimer's. Maybe it's from having nothing to think about. *I* have found you've got to make a goal for yourself, even if you're living in a little corner of a little room." She swept a hand outward, gesturing at her half of the small room, furnished with an antique writing desk, a few family photographs, an armchair, a TV, a stack of books from a local library.

For months her chief occupation had been the Linda Manor Players and the cabaret. It had been a mountain of work. She'd assembled about thirty amateur singers, dancers, and actors. She couldn't find enough residents to fill all the standup parts, so she recruited members of the staff, also the nursing home hairdresser and the hairdresser's husband. And like her father before her, she turned to the churches and shanghaied an Episcopal minister and several members of a local Baptist church into the company.

Eleanor had to make painful concessions. The actors would read their parts. "If I'd insisted on memorizing, I couldn't have gotten a corporal's guard." It wasn't easy staging a play when you didn't have a stage and half of your cast was in wheelchairs and the other half was always too busy to make rehearsals. Although she scolded and cajoled, she hadn't managed to get everyone together at any one of the rehearsals—not until the dress rehearsal, which, she didn't mind saying, was pretty ragged. She also had to fire the first piano player she engaged. Several times lately she'd threatened to cancel the whole thing. "I should never have tried to do something this ambitious," Eleanor said, back upstairs in her room. But there was a lot of color in her face, not all of it from the rouge on her cheeks. She was smiling.

"You say I inveigled you into Eleanor's play," Lou said from his chair by the window.

"You got me into . . ." Joe began to say, his voice on the verge of a bellow.

"Joe, the word you like to use, I don't like to use it. Bullshit. *I* got inveigled just by suggesting a few jokes to her."

They'd been having this same discussion for a few weeks now. "I did many stupid things," Joe said. "But this play of Ellen-er's . . ."

"Oh, you'll do all right," Lou said. "You signed the contract and you gotta live up to it."

"Listen." Joe rose up in bed, pulling back the private curtain to face Lou. "I did high school plays and I did all right. But this script, for Christ's sake, it stinks, huh?"

"Oh, it doesn't stink," Lou said, adding, "I don't have a script. I'm playing it by ear."

In the evening they made their way downstairs, dressed in their costumes—Lou in a large, floppy, snap-brim hat, Joe with a cloth band tied around his head. From the elevator landing all the way down on Sunrise wing, one could hear the babble of the gathering theater crowd.

As the cast assembled in the activity room, Bob looked around at their costumes, the floppy hats, the black gloves, the several fancy dresses, and said, "Oh, boy, oh boy. Excellent."

"I don't want to hear that word," said Eleanor. "Not tonight."

Bob sat in the chorus, grinning at everything, along with Phil and several women in wheelchairs. The major singers and players sat in front of the chorus, in a row of folding chairs across the dining room doorway, in about the same position that Bob and Lou and Joe occupied for pre-meal Stupidvising. This spot now became the stage. The actors faced the dining room, where their audience sat.

At one end of the front row of actors sat Lou and Joe. Joe looked amused and a little embarrassed. Eleanor sat at the other end of the front row, beside the piano and the drummer, who was a nurse's son. The rest of that row were Eleanor's able-bodied, younger ringers: Linda Manor's director of activities, her assistant, an administrative assistant in charge of scheduling, two youngish Baptist friends of Eleanor's, the Baptist minister, who wore a dark suit and would serve as "Mr. Interlocutor," and a nursing supervisor whose pretty soprano equaled in volume the combined voices of the rest of the company and, it must be said, saved most of the musical parts of the show. The company rose, and with sweet and sour notes, the cabaret began.

On a bright and pleasant morning in the springtime
When the birds are sweetly singing in the shade,
There is nothing half so thrilling to the senses
As to see a minstrel troupe to their parade.
Ta ta ta tum,
On they come . . .

The company sat down. Rising, Mr. Interlocutor gestured at the row of actors, saying to the audience, "Ladies and gentlemen, the funmakers of the evening." The audience clapped loudly.

The audience overflowed the dining room. In the back were a number of the actors' relatives—children, grandchildren, a great-grandchild or two, many of them standing, some sitting on the windowsills. The residents in the audience, mainly in wheelchairs, sat at the round dining tables. Most seemed more interested in the hors d'oeuvres than in the show.

Up on the stage—the open patch of gray linoleum floor where the stage should have been—Mr. Interlocutor said to Mr. Charcoal, "Your brother is an author, I believe."

"Oh, yes. Pinky am an author. Is you read his last book?"

"No. What is it?"

"It's pigs. De social life of pigs. It *sho'* am a *swill* book."

One of the residents in the audience said to another, "Well, at least they have a sense of humor." Behind them, though, the younger contingent laughed and laughed. As the show went on, the female residents at one table in the audience discussed the finger foods. Why did the kitchen serve them food you needed teeth to eat? And where were the napkins? But the rest of the audience drowned out most of that conversation. The audience laughed at all the right moments and applauded at the end of every song, dialogue, and skit.

Joe, playing Simon Legree in Eleanor's father's egregious "Uncle Tom's Nabin," fumbled his lines, trying to read his script. Eleanor prompted him, hissing from stage left, and Joe found his voice. "I'll have his blood!" Joe roared, flicking a riding crop over Uncle Tom, Linda Manor's chief of maintenance, who lay snoring on the floor. The third actor in this bit, a retired school principal in a wheelchair with a painful-looking hump, declared, her mordant voice improving the line: "You can't. He's anemic."

Eleanor donned a bonnet, tied its strings under her chin, and remained seated beside the drummer for her solo. "My mother sang this song in my father's revue when I was two and a half years old, but I'm no singer, so I will speak it," she told the audience, and then slipped into character, hunching her shoulders, clasping her hands together, pulling them to her chest, and saying, "I'm an old maid, an old maid. That's what the people say. Although"—she paused, her hands coming forward, palms facing up—"although I'm very fond of men, they never come my way . . ."

Eleanor was the smoothest of the performers, clearly a trained actress acting. But Winifred, in the role of a nagging, weeping wife to a bankrupt ne'er-do-well, was utterly convincing, a natural talent now exposed. Everyone knew Winifred, and she got a big hand when her able-bodied partner in the skit wheeled her out before the audience. Winifred wore a bouffant, curly brown wig, like a headdress, and a satin print dress with perhaps two pounds of costume jewelry around her neck. Her wheelchair had leg extenders on which her swollen feet and legs rested, pointing straight out at the audience. Winifred was huge all over and in outline nearly shapeless, but for all of that she looked regal, like a queen in a peculiar dream. Her voice was very strong. It seemed a pity that she didn't have more lines.

Lou came on near the end of the show, rising and walking slowly on his cane to center stage. Lou didn't use any of Eleanor's father's material. He did three old vaudeville turns remembered from his youth. They were two-man acts. Lou did both voices. "On the way out I met an old friend of mine who just came back from a course in school where he learned all about nature. I said, 'You did? What is nature?' 'Well, I'll tell ya. You plant a sweet potato and it grows, that's nature.' 'Oh, nature is a sweet potato? Ah, you didn't learn nothin.' Tell the people everything you learned.' 'I'll tell them everything we *both* learned. It won't take any longer.'

"Ladies and gentlemen," Lou said at last, "we'll be here tonight, tomorrow night, and probably Saturday night. Provided police and weather conditions permit." The audience laughed uncertainly. "That's all, folks," Lou added, and everybody cheered.

Soon Mr. Interlocutor was saying, "Ladies and gentlemen, the finale by the entire company," and, led by the nursing supervisor's fine, strong soprano, they began, "Ta ta ta tum, on they come . . ." The front row of actors was supposed to stand to sing.

Lou stood up. Beside him, Joe inched himself to the edge of his low metal chair, planted his cane, and started to rise. Many days had passed since he had gone to M&M's or ridden the bike, because of his blister. Joe's arm trembled. He rose a little and then settled back. He tried again. His arm shook as it tried to push him up.

Lou turned and reached down to help, but by then the song was almost over, and Joe waved him away.

permissions

"Bed, Blanket, Window" by Carol Sanford. Copyright © by Carol Sanford.

"Mirrorings" by Lucy Grealy. Copyright © 1993 by *Harper's Magazine*. All rights reserved. Reproduced from the February issue by special permission.

"In Praise of Vanilla" from *A Natural History of the Senses* by Diane Ackerman. Copyright © 1990 by Diane Ackerman. Reprinted by permission of Random House.

"Dora Rewriting Freud: Desiring to Heal" from *The Poetry of Healing: A Doctor's Education in Empathy, Identity, and Desire* by Raphael Campo. Copyright © 1997 by Raphael Campo. Used by permission of W. W. Norton & Company.

Excerpts from *Misgivings* by C. K. Williams. Copyright © 2000 by C. K. Williams. Reprinted by permission of Farrar, Straus and Giroux.

"Last Things" by Debra Spark. Copyright © 1994 *Ploughshares*. Reprinted by permission of Debra Spark.

"A Neurologist's Notebook: A Surgeon's Life" by Oliver Sacks. Reproduced by permission of International Creative Management.

"An Unspoken Art" from *An Unspoken Art* by Lee Gutkind. Copyright © 1997 by Lee Gutkind. Reprinted by permission of Henry Holt and Company.

"Falling into Life" by Leonard Kriegel. Reprinted by permission of The Creative Nonfiction Foundation.

"In Memoriam" from *The Least of These My Brethen* by Daniel D. Baxter, M.D. Reprinted by permission of Harmony Books, a division of Crown Publishers.

"Liferower" by Rebecca McClanahan. Reprinted by permission of The Creative Nonfiction Foundation.

"Intoxicated by My Illness" by Anatole Broyard. Copyright © 1989 by the New York Times Co. Reprinted by permission.

about the editor

Lee Gutkind, founder and editor of the popular journal, *Creative Nonfiction,* has performed as a clown for Ringling Brothers, scrubbed with heart and liver transplant surgeons, wandered the country on a motorcycle, and experienced psychotherapy with a distressed family—all as research for eight books and numerous profiles and essays, including the award-winning "Many Sleepless Nights," an inside chronicle of the world of organ transplantation; "Stuck in Time," which captures the tragedy of childhood mental illness, and most recently, "An Unspoken Art, Profiles of Veterinary Life." University of Southern Illinois Press recently reissued Gutkind's book about major league umpires, *The Best Seat in Baseball, But You Have to Stand!* which *USA Today* called "unprecedented, revealing, startling and poignant."

Former director of the writing program at the University of Pittsburgh and currently professor of English, Lee Gutkind has pioneered the teaching of creative nonfiction, conducting workshops and presenting readings throughout the United States. Also a novelist and filmmaker, Gutkind is director of the Mid-Atlantic Creative Nonfiction Writers Conference at Goucher College in Baltimore.